Integrated Medical Sciences

Integrated Medical Sciences

The Essentials

Shantha Perera   Principal author

University of Wolverhampton, UK

Stephen Anderson

University of Wolverhampton, UK

Ho Leung

Lea Road Medical Practice, Wolverhampton, UK

Rousseau Gama

New Cross Hospital, Wolverhampton, UK

John Wiley & Sons, Ltd

Other Wiley Editorial Offices

John Wiley & Sons Inc., 111 River Street, Hoboken, NJ 07030, USA

Jossey-Bass, 989 Market Street, San Francisco, CA 94103-1741, USA

Wiley-VCH Verlag GmbH, Boschstr. 12, D-69469 Weinheim, Germany

John Wiley & Sons Australia Ltd, 42 McDougall Street, Milton, Queensland 4064, Australia

John Wiley & Sons (Asia) Pte Ltd, 2 Clementi Loop #02-01, Jin Xing Distripark, Singapore 129809

John Wiley & Sons Canada Ltd, 6045 Freemont Blvd, Mississauga, Ontario, L5R 4J3

Wiley also publishes its books in a variety of electronic formats. Some content that appears in print may not be
available in electronic books.

Century Logo Design by Richard J. Pacifico

Library of Congress Cataloging-in-Publication Data

Integrated medical sciences : the essentials / Shantha Perera ... [et al.].
    p. ; cm.
Includes bibliographical references and index.
ISBN 978-0-470-01658-9 (cloth : alk. paper) – ISBN 978-0-470-01659-6 (pbk. : alk. paper)
1. Medical sciences–Case studies. I. Perera, Shantha.
[DNLM: 1. Medicine–Problems and Exercises. WB 18.2 I611 2007]
RC66.I54 2007
616.0076–dc22   2007011330

British Library Cataloguing in Publication Data

A catalogue record for this book is available from the British Library

ISBN 978-0-470-01658-9 (HB)   ISBN 978-0-470-01659-6 (PB)

Typeset in 10.5/12.5pt Minion by Thomson Digital
Printed and bound in Great Britain by Antony Rowe Ltd., Chippenham, Wilts
This book is printed on acid-free paper responsibly manufactured from sustainable forestry
in which at least two trees are planted for each one used for paper production.

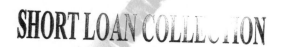

Dedicated to the memory of

Dr Y. S. Perera (1919–2002),

*physician, teacher, beloved father. A guiding light
and source of inspiration that will never
diminish with the passage of time.*

Shantha Perera

Contents

About this book...

This book aims to present the essential concepts and facts of the basic medical sciences through case scenarios involving a group of characters. It is therefore primarily a revision text.

The book is set out in 10 chapters. Chapters 1–8 cover the organ systems that constitute the human body. Chapters 9 and 10 cover the haematological and immune systems, inheritance and the principles of infection.

Each chapter contains clinical scenarios involving common disease conditions affecting the system under consideration. As you read through these disease scenarios you will be introduced to the underlying basic medical science principles: the anatomical, physiological, biochemical, pharmacological and pathological principles and facts relevant to the system.

For example, the chapter on the digestive system involves several scenarios where common disorders involving the different parts/organs of the digestive system are encountered. As you read these scenarios you will be presented with the anatomy, physiology and biochemistry relevant to that particular part of the digestive system. You will also be introduced to the relevant pathophysiology, pharmacology and microbiology. The scientific facts and concepts would be presented in a fully integrated manner in the context of the clinical scenarios.

The clinical scenarios involve a group of characters that appear throughout the book. You will come across them repeatedly as you read through the chapters and will get to know their medical conditions and personalities. This approach, will aid recall and also be useful when you enter the clinical years where you will encounter patients with multiple clinical problems that require an integrated approach.

For students who do not have a clinical training period as part of their program (e.g. BSc/MSc students) the integrated, case-based approach will aid in better understanding of the underlying scientific principles. In addition to aiding recall, the problem-solving approach will stimulate lateral thinking and allow an appreciation of the interrelationships between the various specialties of biomedical science.

The text is suitable as a revision text for:

A. Preclinical UK Medical Students preparing for integrated preclinical examinations

B. Preclinical US and International Medical Students preparing for the USMLE Step 1

C. Clinical Physiology BSc students

D. Biomedical Sciences BSc/MSc students

E. BPharm Students

F. Advanced Nurse Practitioners and other Health Sciences students.

Key features of this book

A. *Case Scenarios* involving a cast of characters that appear throughout the book.

B. *Questions* that require you to think about the contents of the scenario; e.g. interpretation of physical findings, lab results, etc.

C. Case scenarios are followed by a consideration of the relevant underlying scientific principles (e.g. anatomy, physiology, biochemistry, pharmacology, etc.) presented mainly by annotated figures, tables and descriptive text.

D. *Trigger Boxes* showing key facts – you will need to work out the significance of the terms, which can be used for rapid revision.

E. *Tables* containing more detailed information.

F. *Incomplete tables* – you need to complete these – if required by your programme of study – they can also be very useful for rapid revision.

G. *Learning Tasks* that will get you vital additional information if required.

How to use this book

This book requires *active* learning on your part.

Read through the clinical scenarios and get a feel of what is going on. Try to answer the questions that follow the text. These questions are aimed to get you to think about the key concepts 'hidden' within the scenario. Some questions also stimulate further reading.

As you continue reading you will be introduced to the underlying scientific principles and key facts in the form of explanatory passages, annotated figures, and tables. Study these carefully and see how they relate to what's happening to the patient. You will also come across some incomplete tables. The incomplete tables are designed to cover additional, more peripheral information that may be required by some programs of study. For example BSc/MSC biomedicine students may not need the level of anatomical detail as medical or nursing students.

The learning tasks are also designed to widen knowledge. Carrying them out will give you the depth required in some programs.

Study the Trigger tables which cover the major diseases relevant to a given system. These tables, which require active learning, will be useful for rapid revision, for example just prior to an examination.

The book has an associated website, containing MCQs and additional topics–please visit www.wiley.com/go/perera

Acknowledgments

We gratefully acknowledge the comments, corrections, help and advice given by the following individuals.

Ms Jane Astley, *University of Wolverhampton, UK*

Dr Paul Barrow, *University of Wolverhampton UK*

Dr Philip Brammer Russells Hall Hospital, UK

Dr Simon Dunmore *University of Wolverhampton UK*

Dr Rufus Fernando New Cross Hospital, UK

Dr Geoff Frampton *University of Wolverhampton UK*

Dr Jan Martin *University of Wolverhampton UK*

Dr Gillian Pearce *University of Wolverhampton UK*

Dr William Simmons *University of Wolverhampton UK*

Dr James Vickers *University of Wolverhampton UK*

We would also like to thank the following individuals for their invaluable help and patience:

Mrs. Doreen Perera, Mr. Robert Hambrook, Ms. Fiona Woods and Ms. Rachael Ballard

The Authors

List of Abbreviations

Ab	antibody
ACE	angiotensin converting enzyme
ACEI	ACE inhibitors
ACh	acetylcholine
ACL	anterior cruciate ligament
ACTH	adrenocorticotrophic hormone
AD	autosomal dominant
ADA	adenosine deaminase
AF	atrial fibrillation
AFP	alpha- fetoprotein
Ag	antigen
AGIs	alpha-glucosidase inhibitors
AIDS	aquired immunodeficiency syndrome
ALL	acute lymphoblastic leukaemia
ALS	amyotrophic lateral sclerosis
ALT	alanine transaminase
AML	acute myeloid leukaemia
ANA	anti-nuclear antibody
ANP	atrial natriuretic peptide
ANS	autonomic nervous system
APC	antigen presenting cell
aPTT	activated partial thromboplastin time
AR	autosomal recessive
ARDS	adult respiratory distress syndrome
ARF	acute renal failure
ASD	atrial septal defect
ASO	anti streptolysin O
AST	aspartate transaminase
AXR	abdominal X ray
AVM	arteriovenous malformation
AZT	azidothymidine
BCG	Bacille Calmette-Guérin
BMT	bone marrow transplant
BP	blood pressure
BPH	benign prostatic hypertrophy
BPV	benign positional vertigo
CA -125	cancer antigen 125
CA -15-3	cancer antigen 15-3
CABG	coronary artery bypass grafting
CAD	coronary artery disease

C-ANCA	circulating anti neutrophil cytoplasmic antibody
CCK	cholecystokinin
CEA	carcinoembryonic antigen
CF	cystic fibrosis
CGD	chronic granulomatous disease
CHF	congestive heart failure
CIN	cervical epithelial neoplasia
CJD	Creutzfeld-Jakob disease
CLL	chronic lymphatic leukaemia
CM	chylomicrons
CML	chronic myeloid leukaemia
CMV	cytomegalovirus
CN	cranial nerve
CNS	central nervous system
CO	cardiac output
COMT	catechol-o-methyl transferase
COPD	chronic obstructive pulmonary disease
COX	cyclooxygenase
CPK-MP	creatine phosphokinase MB fraction
CREST	(calcinosis, Raynaud's, oesophageal dismobility, sclerodactyl, telangiectasia)
CRF	chronic renal failure
CRH	corticotrophin releasing factor
CSF	cerebro spinal fluid
CT	computer tomography
CVA	costovertebral angle or cerebral vascular accident
CXR	chest X ray
DA	dopamine
DDVAP	desmopressin acetate
DHEA	dehydroepiandrosterone
DIC	disseminated intravascular coagulation
DIP	distal interphalangeal joint
DIT	diiodotyrosine
DKA	diabetic ketoacidosis
DM	diabetes mellitus
DMARD	disease modifying anti-rheumatic drug
DNA	deoxyribonucleic acid
DTR	deep tendon reflexes
DUB	dysfunctional uterine bleeding
DVT	deep vein thrombosis
EDV	end diastolic volume
EF	ejection fraction
EF-2	elongation factor 2
ELISA	enzyme linked immunosorbent assay
EPP	end plate potential

EPSP	excitatory postsynaptic potential
ERPOC	evacuation of retained product of conception
ESR	erythrocyte sedimentation rate
ESV	end systolic volume
FEV1	forced expiratory volume 1
FF	filtration fraction
FFP	fresh frozen plasma
FSH	follicle-stimulating hormone
FT3	tri idothyronine
FTA-ABS	fluorescent treponemal antibody - ABS absorption
FVC	forced vital capacity
G6PD	glucose 6 phosphatase deficiency
GABA	gamma amino butyric acid
GBM	glioblastoma multiforme/glomerular basement membrane
GFR	glomerular filtration rate
GGT	gamma glutyryl transferase
GH	growth hormone
GHIH	growth hormone inhibiting hormone
GHRH	growth hormone releasing hormone
GIFT	gamete intrafallopian transfer
GM-CSF	granulocyte monocyte colony stimulating factor
GN	glomerulonephrtis
GnRH	gonadotrophin releasing hormone
GORD	gastroesophageal reflux disease
GTN	glycerine trinitrate
5HT	5-hydroxytryptamine
5 HIAA	5-Hydroxyindolacetic Acid
HAART	highly active antiretroviral therapy
Hb	haemoglobin
HBcAb	hepatitis B core antibody
HBeAb	hepatitis B e antibody
HBeAg	hepatitis B e antigen
HBsAg	hepatitis B surface antgen
hCG	human chorionic gonadotrophin
HD	Huntington's disease
HDL	high density lipoprotein
hGH	human growth hormone
Hib	haemophilus type B vaccine
HIV	human immunodeficiency virus
HLA	human leucocyte antigen
HONK	hyperosmolar hyperglycaemic non-ketotic coma
HPA	hypothalamus-pituitary-adrenal axis
HPL	human placental lactogen
HPV	human papilloma virus
HRT	hormone replacement treatment

HSV	herpes simplex virus
HTLV	human T cell leukaemia virus
HTN	hypertension
HUS	haemolytic uraemic syndrome
IBD	inflammatory bowel disease
IDDM	insulin dependent diabetes mellitus
IFN	interferon
Ig	immunoglobulin
IGF-	insulin-like growth factor 1
IGT	impaired glucose tolerance
INH	isoniazid
INR	international normalised ratio
IPSP	inhibitory post synaptic potential
IRV	inspiratory reserve volume
ITP	idiopathic thrombocytopaenic purpura
IUGR	intrauterine growth retardation
IUI	Intra-uterine insemination
IVC	inferior vena cava
IVF	In vitro fertilization
JRA	juvenile rheumatoid arthritis
JVD	jugular venous distension
JVP	Jugular venous pressure
LAD	left anterior decending
LBBB	left bundle branch block
LDH	lactate dehydrogenase
LDL	low density lipoprotein
LFT	liver function test
LH	lutenizing hormone
LLQ	left lower quadrant
LMN	lower motor neuron
LSD	lysergic acid diethylamide
LV	left ventricle
LVH	left ventricular hypertrophy
MAOI	monoamine oxidase inhibitors
MCH	mean corpuscular haemoglobin
MHC	major histocompatibilty antigen
MCHC	mean cell haemoglobin concentration
MD	macular degeneration
MEN	multiple endocrine neoplasia
MI	myocardial infarction
MIBG	metaiodobenzylguanadine scan
MIT	monoidotryosine
MMR	measles mumps rubella
MPTP	methylphenyltetrahydropyridine
MRCP	magnetic resonance cholangiopancreatography

MRI	magnetic resonance imaging
MS	multiple sclerosis
MSAFP	maternal serum AFP
MSH	melanocyte stimulating hormone
MVP	mitral valve prolapse
NAFLD	non-alcholic fatty acid liver disease
NE	noradrenaline
NGU	non-gonococcal urethritis
NMJ	neuromuscular junction
NSAID	non steroidal anti inflammatory drugs
NSTEMI	non ST elevation myocardial infarctions
OGD	oesophagogastroduedenoscopy
OPV	oral polio vaccine
PAF	platelet activating factor
PAH	para aminohippuric acid
PAN	polyarteritis nodosa
P-ANCA	perinuclear anti neutrophil cytoplasmic antibody
PAP smear	Papanicolaou smear
PCL	posterior cruciate ligament
PCOS	polycystic ovarian syndrome
PDA	patent ductus arteriosus
PE	pulmonary embolism
PEFR	peak expiratory flow rate
PID	pelvic inflammatory disease
PK	pyruvate kinase
PMN	polymorphonuclear leucocyte
PNH	paroxysmal nocturnal haemoglubinuria
PNS	parasympathetic nervous system/peripheral nervous system
PPD	purified protein derivative
PPI	proton pump inhibitor
PPP	pentose-phosphate pathway
PROM	premature rupture of membranes
PSA	prostate specific antigen
PSVT	paroxysmal supraventricular tachycardia
PT	prothrombin time
PTCA	percutaeneous transluminal coronary angioplasty
PTH	parathyroid hormone
PVB	premature ventricular beat
PVC	premature ventricular tachycardia
RA	rheumatoid arthritis
RBBB	right bundle branch block
RBC	red blood cell
RBF	renal blood flow
RDS	respiratory distress syndrome
RF	rheumatic fever

RhoGAM	Rh Immune Globulin
RPR	rapid plasma reagin
RR	respiratory rate
RSV	respiratory syncytial virus/ rous sarcoma virus
RT	reverse transcriptase
RTA	renal tubular acidosis
RUQ	right upper quadrant
RV	residual volume
RV	right ventricle
RVH	right ventricular hypertrophy
SCC	squamous cell carcinoma antigen
SCID	severe combined immunodeficiency
SHBG	sex hormone binding globulin
SIADH	syndrome of inappropriate anti diuretic hormone
SLE	systemic lupus erythymatosus
SMA	superior mesenteric artery
SNS	sympathetic nervous system
SRS-A	slow reacting substance A
SSRI	selective serotonin reuptake inhibitor
SV	stroke volume
SVC	superior vena cava
SVT	supraventricular tachycardia
T max	transport maximum
TAH-BSO	total abdominal hysterectomy & bilateral salphingo-oophorectomy
TB	tuberculosis
TCR	T cell receptor
TG	triglyceride
Th cell	T helper cell
TIA	transient ischaemic attack
TLC	total lung capacity
TMP-SMX	trimethoprim sulphamethoxazole
TNA	tranexemic acid
TNF	tumor necrosis factor
TOA	tuboovarian abscess
TOF	tracheo-oesophageal fistula
t-PA	tissue type plasminogen activator
TPR	total peripheral resistance
TRH	thyrotropin-releasing hormone
TS	tumor suppressor
TSH	thyroid stimulating hormone
TSST-1	toxic shock syndrome toxin 1
TTP	thrombotic thrombocytopaenic purpura
TV	tidal volume
TZD	thiazolidinedione
UDPGR	UDP-glucuronyl transferase

UMN	upper motor neurons
UOS	upper oesophageal sphincter
UTI	urinary tract infection
V/Q ratio	ventilation perfusion ratio
VC	vital capacity
VDRL	venereal disease research laboratory
VIP	vasoactive intestinal peptide
VLDL	very low density lipoprotein
VMA	vanillylmandelic acid
VSD	ventricular septal defect
VT	ventricular tachycardia
VWD	Von Willebrand Disease
VWF	Von Willebrand factor
VZV	varicella zoster virus
WBC	white blood cell

The Sickalott family tree

1

The respiratory system

Learning strategy

In this chapter we will consider the essential 'must know' facts and concepts of the respiratory system. Our main strategy would involve an exploration of these key principles by following several clinical scenarios.

The first scenario, an asthma attack will introduce us to the anatomy of the respiratory system. A consideration of the pathophysiology of asthma, will lead to a review of the immune system and the mechanism of Type 1 hypersensitivity.

Breathing difficulties will lead us to consider the mechanism of breathing and lung compliance. Lung volumes and capacities will be discussed as we consider the lung function tests of the asthmatic patient. We will also review the key drugs used in asthma treatment.

A second scenario – COPD – leads us to a consideration of acidosis and alkalosis. We will also discuss some key respiratory infections and the important concepts of V/Q mismatch and dead space. Finally we will consider gas exchange, oxygen and carbon dioxide saturation curves and the central and peripheral control of respiration.

Throughout, we will also consider the pathophysiological mechanisms of several key disease states involving the respiratory system, which will, in addition to highlighting the key pathophysiological principles, further reinforce basic principles of anatomy, physiology and pharmacology relevant to the respiratory system.

Try to answer the questions and try to complete the Learning Tasks. The Trigger Boxes should be used as a guide for further reading and revision. At the end of this chapter you should have a sound understanding of the key facts and concepts underlying the respiratory system.

Integrated Medical Sciences by Shantha Perera, Stephen Anderson, Ho Leung and Rousseau Gama
© 2007 John Wiley & Sons, Ltd ISBN: 978470016589 (HB) 978470016596 (PB)

Zoe's breathing difficulties . . .

It happened again on Boxing Day. Around 5pm Zoe was sitting on her bed reading when she started to become breathless. Breathing was always her 'problem' and Zoe couldn't understand it.

'After all it's supposed to be such a simple thing to do isn't it?' she had asked Mary. 'It's supposed to be automatic isn't it? I mean you just breathe in and out. So why is it such an effort sometimes?'

Zoe took a puff out of her blue inhaler. She wondered if her problems had something to do with the fact that she had been a premature baby and that that she had to be delivered at 33 weeks, by caesarean section.

'Maybe my lungs weren't developed properly' she thought.

What is in Zoe's blue inhaler?

Although Zoe was a premature baby, she didn't have any problems and grew into a healthy child. Had she been born around, say, 26 weeks she would have had serious problems because her respiratory system would have been underdeveloped.

So, let us begin by reviewing the key stages in the development of the respiratory system. First, in terms of origins, the epithelium of the nasopharynx, trachea, bronchi, bronchioles and alveoli are derived from endoderm. The associated cartilage and muscle are mesodermal in origin.

You are expected to know the embryological origins of key anatomical structures. Construct a table listing the main derivatives of endoderm, ectoderm and mesoderm.

So what are the key embryological events in the development of the respiratory system? The respiratory system starts off as an outgrowth of the foregut. In the 4th week the oesophagotracheal septum separates the foregut into the respiratory diverticulum (lung bud) and oesophagus (Figure 1.1). The bud elongates and then branches into two. Each of these two new buds will become the primary bronchus of each lung.

What happens if the diverticulum fails to separate completely from the foregut
What is a TOF (tracheo-oesophageal fistula)?

The left lung bud develops into two secondary bronchi and eventually forms two lobes; the right bud forms three secondary bronchi and three lobes. The tertiary bronchi create the bronchopulmonary segments.

Gas exchange between blood and air in the primitive alveoli is possible in the seventh month of gestation. Lung growth after birth is mainly due to an increase in the number of respiratory bronchioles and alveoli and not due to an increase in size of alveoli. New alveoli are formed for at least 10 years of postnatal life.

What do we mean by the term 'gas exchange'?

Before birth, the lungs are filled with fluid containing surfactant mainly made up of dipalmitoyl phosphatidylcholine, which is produced by type II epithelial cells. When

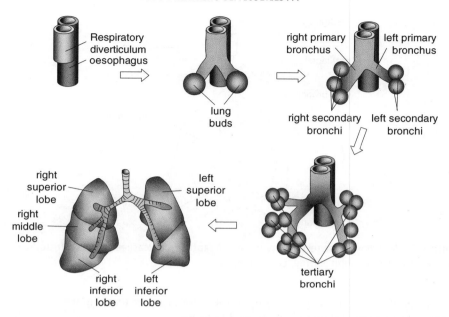

Figure 1.1 Development of the respiratory system. Adapted from Tortora and Grabowski (2003), principles of Anatomy and Physiology, 10th edition, John Wiley & Sons Inc. p.842

respiration begins, lung fluid is reabsorbed but leaves a surfactant coating. If Zoe was born around 26 weeks, her surfactant levels would have been low. She would suffer from respiratory distress syndrome (RDS). Her lungs would be difficult to expand and during deflation her alveoli would collapse. Surfactant decreases the alveolar surface tension and helps the alveoli to expand more easily.

What are type I and II pneumocytes? Where do you find them?
Mothers of premature babies are treated with steroids. Why?
What treatment can be given to a 28-week premature baby having difficulty inflating its lungs?

Trigger box **Respiratory distress syndrome (RDS)**

Deficiency of surfactant causes alveolar collapse and poor gas exchange.
Majority of infants born before 28 weeks develop RDS within 4 hours of birth.
Features: Tachypnoea, cyanosis, diaphragm, subcostal and intercostal retraction, grunting.
CXR: Reticulogranular appearance with air bronchograms.
Treatment: Glucocorticoids to mother, exogenous surfactant, oxygen, continuous positive airway pressure (CPAP), artificial ventilation.

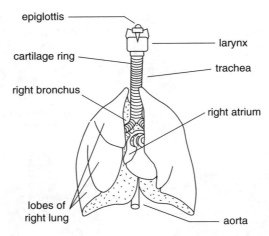

Figure 1.2 Anatomy of the respiratory system. Adapted from Mackean (1969), Introduction to Biology, 4th edition, John Murray, London, p.69.

Next let us consider the gross anatomy of the respiratory system. Figure 1.2 shows the important anatomical structures you need to know.

Note that the right lung has three lobes; the left has two. Each lung lobe is made up of bronchopulmonary segments. Label the oblique and horizontal fissures. The right main bronchus is straighter and shorter than the left main bronchus. This helps to explain why Zoe's brother John, at age 4, got a small peanut stuck in the right main bronchus when he inhaled it.

When Zoe's great-uncle Arthur suffered from a really nasty bout of pulmonary tuberculosis the surgeons had to remove several of his bronchopulmonary segments. This was not too difficult because each bronchopulmonary segment is served by its own arteries and vein and is partitioned from other segments by connective tissue.

 Define what is meant by the terms (a) 'respiratory bronchiole' and (b) 'terminal bronchiole'.

Let us look at the other main structures that make up the respiratory system. Important structures to know include the nasopharynx, oropharynx, larynx, glottis and trachea. The blood supply of the lungs consists of the pulmonary arteries that run with the airways, the bronchial arteries that branch off from the aorta, and the pulmonary veins that run in the connective tissue septa.

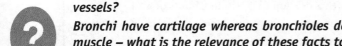

What kind of blood (oxygenated, deoxygenated) is found in these different vessels?

Bronchi have cartilage whereas bronchioles do not. They both have smooth muscle – what is the relevance of these facts to asthma?

Lung connective tissue contains lots of elastic tissue – what is the significance of this elasticity?

The lungs are covered by visceral pleura. This is separated from the parietal pleura which covers the inside of the chest wall by the interpleural space.

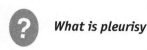 **What is pleurisy**

Trigger box   Pleural effusions

Transudate: (protein <30 g/L; LDH <200 iu/l):
Congestive heart failure (CHF), hypothyroidism, nephrotic syndrome
Exudate: (protein >30 g/L; LDH >200 iu/l):
Pneumonia, carcinoma, tuberculosis (TB), pulmonary infarct.
Can detect clinically if >500mL; by CXR >300mL.
Findings: Reduced chest movements, stony dull percussion, decreased breath sounds, reduced vocal resonance. Blunting of costophrenic angle on CXR.
Treatment: drain exudates, treat underlying cause of transudate.
Sclerosing agents to reduce recurrent malignant pleural effusions.

Three years ago Dr Smith, Zoe's GP, had told her that she had asthma. Zoe was also told that this was related to her tendency to suffer from allergies. Also, colds, he stated, can lead to an asthma attack – and she got plenty of those especially in winter.

'The problem is with your immune system' Dr Smith said.

'What's wrong with my immune system?' Zoe asked. 'Isn't it supposed to defend me, zap these nasty bugs?'

'Your immune system is reacting inappropriately to certain antigens' replied Dr Smith and then went on to explain how her immune system was causing her asthma and allergic reactions.

This leads us to introduce the basics of the immune system, which needs to be understood in order to appreciate the pathophysiology of Zoe's asthma. This important system will be considered in detail in Chapter 10 but Figure 1.3 will help to explain what is meant by appropriate and inappropriate immune responses.

Note the central role of the Th cell and the Tc response that can eliminate viruses. This is an *appropriate* immune response. Type I hypersensitivity on the other hand, is an *inappropriate* immune response brought about by the generation of IgE reaginic antibodies against allergens, which leads to mast cell degranulation and the release of mediators that give rise to inflammation and the asthmatic symptoms. Goodpasture's syndrome is a type II hypersensitivity reaction affecting the lung. A type III disease affecting the lung is hypersensitivity pneumonitis and an important type IV hypersensitivity disease affecting the lung is tuberculosis.

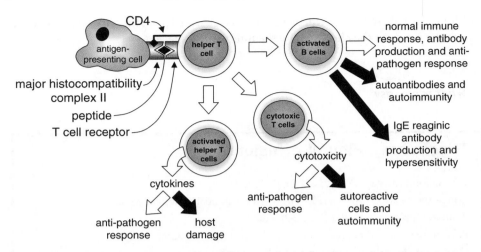

Figure 1.3   Appropriate (open arrows) and inappropriate (closed arrows) immune responses

---

Trigger box   **Hypersensitivity reactions**

Type I
  IgE.
  Primary and secondary mediators from mast cells, basophils.
  Asthma, allergic rhinitis, eczema, urticaria, food allergies, systemic anaphylaxis.

Type II
  Cyotoxic.
  IgG against cell surface antigens – complement-mediated damage.
  Blood group incompatabilities in transfusion, autoimmune haemolytic anaemia (AHA),
  erythroblastosis fetalis, Goodpasture's syndrome.

Type III
  Antigen/antibody (Ag/Ab) complexes – complement activation, neutrophil infiltration.
  Arthus reaction, serum sickness, vasculitis, glomerulonephritis, systemic lupus
  erythematosus (SLE), rheumatoid arthritis (RA), hypersensitivity pneumonitis.

Type IV
  Cell mediated.
  Th1 cells release cytokines – macrophage, T-cell activation –tissue damage.
  Contact dermatitis, TB.

Trigger box **Tuberculosis**

Primary TB – usually lung; usually asymptomatic.
Reactivation leads to post-primary TB (most cases of symptomatic TB), miliary TB.
Findings: Ghon complex (caseating lesions in lymph nodes + granuloma).
Kidney most common site of extrapulmonary TB.
Features: Malaise, anorexia, weight loss, fever, cough, haemoptysis, mucoid, purulent sputum.
Investigations: CXR, ZN stain, Lowenstein–Jensen culture, Mantoux test.
Mantoux positive 5–15 mm in 48–72 h indicates infection and/or bacille Calmette–Guérin (BCG) vaccination.
BCG reduces TB development by 50%.
Treatment: Rifampicin, isoniazid (INH), pyrazinamide, ethambutol.
Pyridoxine to reduce INH neurotoxicity.

 List common allergens

 Can you list the main pathogens responsible for 'colds'?

Trigger box **Hypersensitivity pneumonitis**

A type III hypersensitivity reaction secondary to inhaled organic material (e.g. mouldy hay spores).
Examples: Farmers' lung, bird fanciers' lung.
Findings: Thick alveolar walls, granulomas with histiocytes and plasma cells. Fibrosis in chronic.
Examination: Bilateral crackles.
Diagnosis: CT, lung biopsy.
Treatment: Antigen avoidance, steroids, immunosuppressants.

What are pneumoconioses?

Figure 1.4 shows the mechanism of type I hypersensitivity that is responsible for the pathology of Zoe's acute allergic asthma attack. Note that antigen-binding to IgE stimulates mast cells to release pre-synthesized primary mediators. Synthesis and subsequent release of secondary mediators involve the activation of arachidonic acid and the synthesis and release of prostaglandins and thromboxanes through

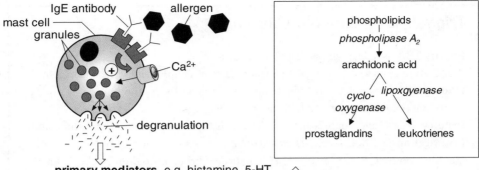

primary mediators, e.g. histamine, 5-HT.
secondary mediators, e.g. prostaglandins.

Figure 1.4 Type 1 hypersensitivity*

Table 1.1 Key primary mediators and their effects

Mediator	Characteristics and effects
Histamine	Basic amine stored in granules of mast cells and basophils. Contracts non-vascular smooth muscle, vasodilatation, increased vascular permeability, enhanced mucus secretion, prostaglandin secretion in the lung, chemokinesis
Serotonin	Increased vascular permeability, smooth muscle contraction
ECF A	Eosinophil chemotaxis
NCF-A	Neutrophil chemotaxis

cyclooxygenase pathway and leukotrienes C4 and D4 (termed slow reacting substance of anaphylaxis (SRS-A)) through the lipoxygenase pathway.

 What is anaphylaxis? Can you describe the mechanisms underlying systemic anaphylaxis? How is this condition treated?

At the time of her diagnosis, Zoe had been given a skin prick test to confirm her allergic status. She was inoculated with a series of allergens including grass pollen and dust mite extracts. She got a classic wheal and flare reaction after 20 minutes but was surprised when the reaction reappeared around 5 hours later. Immediate reactions occur within minutes of allergen exposure and are mediated principally by the mast cell granule contents (primary mediators). Some 5–8 hours after the immediate reaction has subsided, a second reaction – the late-phase reaction – occurs due to the release of additional secondary mediators including cytokines. Tables 1.1 and 1.2 show the key

---

*Note that cross-linking of IgE by allergen leads to receptor cross-linkage. This leads to a transient elevation of cAMP, activation of protein tyrosine kinases, methylation of membrane phospholipids and an influx of calcium which causes fusion of granules with plasma membrane and release of primary mediators into extracellular environment. Secondary mediators are synthesized.

Table 1.2   Key secondary mediators and their effects

Mediator	Characteristics and effects
Cytokines	Stimulate and amplify Th2 cell responses (IL-4, IL-13), promote eosinophil production and activation (IL-3, IL-5, GM-CSF) and promote inflammation (TNF-α).
Prostaglandin E_2	Causes vasodilatation and potentiates increased vascular permeability produced by histamine.
Leukotrienes C_4 and D_4	Causes smooth muscle contraction, increased vascular permeability and mucus secretion.
Platelet-activating factor	Synthesized from phospholipid. Causes platelet and neutrophil activation, increased vascular permeability and smooth muscle contraction.
Major basic protein and eosinophil peroxidase	Triggers histamine release from mast cells. Tissue damage.
Bradykinin	Nonapeptide formed from kininogen. Causes vasodilatation, increased vascular permeability and stimulation of pain nerve endings.

Th2, T helper 2; IL, interleukin; GM-CSF, granulocyte–macrophage colony-stimulating factor; TNF-α, tumour necrosis factor-α.

primary and secondary mediators that lead to the inflammatory reaction seen in type I hypersensitivity.

Cytokines are small proteins (5–20 kDa) that are released from cells and act in a similar way as hormones, affecting cellular behaviour. Cytokines allow cells of the immune system to communicate with each other to modulate immune responses. Cytokines are important in mediating many different types of immune responses. Table 1.3 shows the functions of some key cytokines.

Table 1.3   Some key cytokines and their function

Cytokine	Function
IL-1	Stimulates T- and B-cell proliferation and is a pyrogen
IL-2	Stimulates T- and B-cell proliferation and activates natural killer cells
IL-3	Stimulates B memory cells
IL-4	Stimulates plasma cell formation, IgE synthesis and activates B cells
IL-5	Stimulates plasma cell secretion of IgA and IgM, stimulates B cells and eosinophils
IL-6	Induces B-cell differentiation into plasma cells and induces T-cell proliferation and activation
IFN-α	Inhibits viral replication
IFN-β	Inhibits viral replication
IFN-γ	Stimulates monocytes and macrophages and decreases viral replication
TNF-α	Cytotoxic to tumour cells, cachexia
TNF-β	Cytotoxic and increase phagocytosis

Describe the following terms as applied to cytokine action:

Autocrine
Paracrine
Endocrine
Redundancy
Antagonism
Pleiotrophy
Synergy.

What are the four signs of inflammation?
Which cells are found in sites of acute and chronic inflammation?
Can you define the following: triggers, inducers, intrinsic and extrinsic asthma.

The 'blue' inhaler didn't seem to work for Zoe and she knew what this meant. She was heading for another major asthma attack. Zoe called out to Mary around 7pm. Mary heard her and raced upstairs to find Zoe breathing rapidly, gasping for breath and wheezing. She was sitting at her desk, all hunched up; she could barely speak.

What is the normal respiratory rate for young adults?

Mary called out to John who took one look at Zoe and decided to take her to the Emergency Doctor. Since both John and Mary had been drinking, they had to call a taxi! Zoe was breathing with great difficulty. This distressing scene leads us to consider the mechanics of breathing shown in Figure 1.5.

Note that during inspiration as the chest wall expands (external intercostals) and the diaphragm moves down the two pleurae are moved apart. This causes a more negative

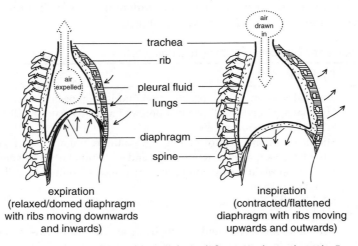

Figure 1.5 The mechanism of breathing. Adapted from Mackean (1969), Introduction to Biology, 4th edition, John Murray, London, p.101.

intrapleural pressure (subatmospheric) to develop. This increase in negative intra-pleural pressure overcomes the natural elasticity (elastic recoil) of the lungs and the surface tension of the inner alveoli lining and the lungs inflate, the negative alveolar pressure drawing air into the lungs. Intercostal nerves innervate the intercostal muscles and the diaphragm is innervated by the phrenic nerve (C3, C4, C5).

Why is a head injury that causes damage to spinal cord above C3, C4 or C5 potentially fatal?

The accessory muscles, sclani, sternocleidomastoids and pectoralis are used in forced inspiration. Remember how Zoe is sitting during her acute asthma attack – she is utilizing her accessory muscles.

The diaphragm is the most important structure involved in breathing. In severe asthmatics, airway obstruction causes air trapping, which tends to hyperinflate the lungs. This causes a barrel-shaped thoracic cavity and a flattening of the diaphragm, which impairs its movement during breathing and leads to shortness of breath.

Some years later Max, Debbie's boyfriend was rushed into the ED after being stabbed in the chest. His left lung collapsed because air was getting into the pleural cavity and was unable to leave because his shirt was stuck to his chest. This is called a tension pneumo-thorax and a chest tube had to be inserted to remove the trapped air and reinflate his lung.

Describe other types of pneumothorax.
Define atelectasis.

Let us now consider the important lung feature of compliance. Compliance is a measure of how expandable the lungs are for a given change in pressure. Zoe's lung compliance is nearly normal. On the other hand Ted, Grandma Irene's brother living down the street who suffers from emphysema has an increased lung compliance. Figure 1.6 shows compliance in different conditions and how compliance can be calculated.

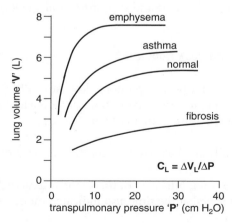

$$C_L = \Delta V_L / \Delta P$$

Figure 1.6 Compliance. Adapted from Berne and Levy (1996) Principles of Physiology, 3rd edition, Mosby

Why does kyphoscoliosis reduce compliance?

The Emergency Doctor listened to Zoe's lungs; she was very wheezy. Zoe's pulse was also checked, which was found to be 109 beats/minute (bpm). Her blood oxygen saturation (O_2 sats) was 78 per cent. Zoe was given nebulized salbutamol. After 5 minutes Zoe was able to talk in complete sentences. Her wheezing was less noticeable and her O_2 sats had gone up to 95 per cent.

What caused the wheezing?
What is the normal oxygen saturation in arterial blood?
Why was Zoe tachycardic?
What is pulsus paradoxus?

On the following Tuesday Mary took a rather reluctant Zoe to see Dr Smith their family doctor. Zoe didn't understand why she had to go, as she was feeling fine. Mary disagreed: Zoe's asthma appeared to be worsening.

Dr Smith asked about her allergies and Zoe mentioned that her asthma was worse after dusting and that she suffered with hay fever in the summer. Zoe also mentioned that her asthma was worse at night and that she would cough and sometimes get wheezy.

Exercise, especially in the cold also made it worse. Zoe then added that she had been suffering from a bad cold 3 days prior to the last big attack.

Dr Smith carried out a full respiratory examination and found Zoe to be tachypnoeic, with a respiration rate of 26 breaths/min and a pulse of 92 bpm. Zoe's ability to expand her chest was checked and found to be normal, but percussion revealed a hyper-resonance and auscultation, some minor wheezing.

Dr Smith then carried out three peak flow readings, which revealed a best of 420 L/min. He reviewed Zoe's file and noted that a spirometry examination carried out 6 months ago had indicated a FEV_1 of 2.4 L and a FEV_1/FVC ratio of 61%. (Figure 1.7 shows the important lung volumes and capacities, and the legend defines the terms commonly used.)

How do you carry out a peak flow test?

At the surgery Zoe showed a peak expiratory flow rate (PEFR) of 420. PEFR is the maximum flow achieved in one forced expiration. PEFR is a useful clinical tool to assess the degree of airway obstruction, particularly in asthma.

    List the key conditions that lead to a decrease of peak flow.

Dr Smith also noted an eosinophilia in a routine blood test carried out around 6 months ago. A chest X-ray performed at the time also indicated moderate hyperinflation.

What is the role of the eosinophil in asthma?

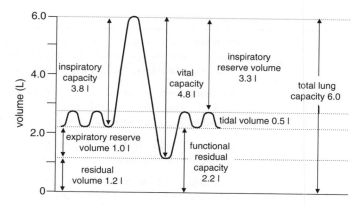

Figure 1.7 Lung volumes and capacities

Lung volumes

Tidal volume, TV: Volume of a single breath, usually at rest.

Inspiratory reserve volume, IRV: Volume that can be inspired beyond a restful inspiration.

Expiratory reserve volume, ERV: Volume that can be expired beyond a restful expiration.

Residual volume, RV: Volume remaining in the lungs after a maximum expiration. This volume keeps the alveoli inflated.

FEV_1 is the volume of gas expelled in first second.

Lung capacities

Total lung capacity: Sum of all the respiratory volumes and residual volume.

$TLC = FRC + IC = VC + RV$

Vital capacity, VC: The vital capacity is the maximum volume, which can be ventilated, in a single breath. $VC = IRV + TV + ERV$. VC varies with gender, age, and build. Measuring VC helps to diagnose respiratory disorders, and is a benchmark for judging the effectiveness of treatment.

Functional residual capacity, FRC: Volume of gas left in the lungs at end of quiet expiration.

Inspiratory capacity: Tidal volume plus inspiratory reserve volume.

Forced vital capacity, FVC: Total volume of expired gas, similar to vital capacity but measured during forced expiration.

Dr Smith then reviewed Zoe's medication. She was on the 'brown' inhaler and was also advised to use the 'blue' inhaler when required. She was also on oral steroids. So, let us now look at the drugs Zoe is using. Table 1.4 shows the main drugs used in asthma.

Why would you have to be careful about prescribing (a) aspirin and (b) beta blockers to asthmatic patients?

What are the main side effects of chronic corticosteroid use?

Describe the Step 1–4 treatment strategies in asthma.

Table 1.4 The main drugs used in asthma

Beta agonists	Salbutamol, albuterol, salmeterol (long acting). They relax airway smooth muscles (via β2 adrenoceptors). Adverse effect: tachycardia (via β1 adrenoceptors).
Corticosteroids	Beclomethasone, prednisolone. They prevent production of leukotrienes from arachidonic acid by blocking phospholipase A2. Drug of choice in status asthmaticus
Antileukotrienes	Zileuton – blocks synthesis of lipoxygenase Zafirlukast – blocks leukotriene receptors
Methylxanthines	Theophylline – bronchodilation by inhibiting phosphodiesterase involved in degrading cAMP
Muscarinic antagonists	Ipratropium – blocks muscarinic receptors preventing bronchoconstriction
Cromolyn (cromoglycate)	Prevents release of mediators from mast cells. Effective only as prophylactic
Anti IgE-monoclonal antibody	Neutralizes IgE

Grandma's bad chest...

With the Christmas and New Year holidays over, the Sickalotts returned to their usual routines. Zoe's wheezing was much less pronounced. Things however took a turn for the worse in the bungalow down the road.

Grandma Irene suffered from chronic obstructive pulmonary disease (COPD) and was under the care of Dr Blunt at Hope Hospital. Dr Blunt was also looking after Ted, Irene's brother who was also suffering from COPD. For the last few months Grandma Irene was finding it harder and harder to breathe. But not being one to complain, she had carried on with her routines, which mainly centred on looking after Albert. However, her cough was getting worse and she became breathless on minimal exertion. During Mary's daily visit, on the 8th of January, Albert told Mary that Irene's coughing was getting a lot worse and that she might have a raised temperature. Mary wanted to take Irene to see Dr Smith. Irene declined, stating that she always got like this in the winter. It was no big deal.

Around midnight that same day, John and Mary were woken up by the telephone ringing incessantly. On the other end of the line was a rather shaky Albert saying that Irene had taken a turn for the worse.

John and Mary rushed over to the bungalow. Irene was sitting in her chair in the living room, attached to her oxygen, with Albert standing next to her and looking very distressed. John called an ambulance and the paramedics arrived 10 minutes later. They found Irene gasping for breath. She looked cyanotic and was using her accessory muscles for breathing. Irene was given nebulized salbutamol and taken to hospital.

At the hospital Irene was examined by one of the duty doctors. He noted the mild cyanosis, the jugular venous distension (JVD) and end expiratory wheezing. He also noted high-pitched bronchial sounds on the left side, crackles and dullness to percussion. Irene's chest showed moderate hyperinflation and her nicotine-stained fingers were noted to be clubbed. Her respiration rate was 45 bpm, her BP was 160/95 and she had a temperature of 39°C. Irene was responsive only to repeated verbal commands. Her treatment started with nebulized salbutamol, i.v. steroids and i.v. ampicillin.

What is JVD?

What is the most likely cause of Irene's increased temperature?

What is the significance of dullness to percussion, high pitched bronchial sounds and finger clubbing?

What is the significance of mentioning Irene's nicotine stained fingers?

Why was Irene treated with ampicillin? What is the mechanism of action of ampicillin?

The duty doctor ordered some arterial blood gases (ABGs), which indicated hypoxaemia, hypercapnia (hypercarbia) and mild respiratory acidosis. A chest X-ray was also ordered.

You should be able to explain the mechanisms involved in respiratory acidosis and alkalosis. Respiratory acidosis is seen when arterial $PaCO_2$ rises above normal (e.g. in Irene's COPD when ventilation was impaired). Conversely, overbreathing, such as during Zoe's acute asthma attack, can cause more CO_2 to be blown off, giving rise to a respiratory alkalosis. Table 1.5 shows the causes of respiratory and metabolic acidosis and alkalosis and also shows the compensatory reactions.

Table 1.5 Acidosis and alkalosis

Condition	Causes	Compensatory mechanism
Respiratory acidosis	Increased $PaCO_2$ and decreased pH due to hypoventilation caused by any lung, neuromuscular or physical cause of respiratory failure.	Increased renal excretion of H^+ ions and increased reabsorption of HCO_3^- ions.
Respiratory alkalosis	Decreased $PaCO_2$ and increased pH due to hyperventilation.	Decreased renal excretion of H^+ ions and decreased reabsorption of HCO_3^- ions.
Metabolic acidosis	Decreased HCO_3^- ion concentration and decreased pH caused by excessive HCO_3^- ion loss or increased H^+ production.	Hyperventilation to increase CO_2 excretion and reduce carbonic acid concentration.
Metabolic alkalosis	Increased HCO_3^- ion concentration and increased pH caused by excessive H^+ ion loss.	Hypoventilation to reduce CO_2 excretion and increase carbonic acid concentration.

What are the typical arterial blood gas findings in (a) acute asthma and (b) acute COPD?

  List other causes that lead to respiratory acidosis and alkalosis.

By next morning, Irene was much better. The doctor noted her sputum pot and requested a sputum culture. He also requested lung function tests which revealed a FEV$_1$ of 1.1 L and a FEV$_1$/FVC ratio of 43 per cent.

Irene, Ted and Zoe suffer from obstructive lung diseases. In these diseases the FEV$_1$/FVC ratio is <80 per cent, in contrast to restrictive diseases where the ratio is >80 per cent.

Trigger box   Key obstructive and restrictive lung diseases

1. *Obstructive lung diseases*

(FEV$_1$/FVC <80%; increased TLC; increased FRC; increased RV).
Chronic bronchitis.
Emphysema.
Asthma.
Bronchiectasis.

2. *Restrictive lung diseases*

(FEV$_1$/FVC >80%; decreased VC; decreased TLC).
Sarcoidosis.
Diffuse interstitial pulmonary fibrosis.
Scoliosis.
Neuromuscular disease (e.g. polio).
Myasthenia gravis.

Trigger box   Diffuse interstitial pulmonary fibrosis

Most common restrictive lung disease.
More common in the elderly.
Pathology: Thick alveolar walls – cystic spaces.
Findings: Shallow rapid breathing, cough.
Reticular pattern/honeycomb pattern on CXR (in severe disease).
Treatment: Supportive, steroids.
What is the aetiology of this disease?

Trigger box   Sarcoidosis

Cause unknown.

Multisystemic disease, most common extrapulmonary manifestations: skin/ocular abnormalities.

Female > male, Afro-Caribbeans > Caucasians, 20–40s,

Findings: Restrictive lung disease; erythema nodosum; lupus pernio; hypercalcaemia; uveitis; uviparotid fever; arythmias; cardiomyopathy; cranial nerve palsies; arthralgias; granulomas (non-caseating); cell-mediated immune depression.

Investigations: CXR (bilateral hilar adenopathy), transbronchial biopsy, angiotensin-converting enzyme (ACE) (increased with disease activity/responds to treatment).

Treatment: Steroids, immunosuppressants.

Trigger box   Cystic fibrosis (CF)

Autosomal recessive (AR).

1:2000.

Mutations in *CFTR* – main delta F508.

Defective Cl^- channel.

Features: Viscous secretions – bronchiectasis, obstructive lung disease; meconium ileus; diabetes mellitus.

Pseudomonas aeruginosa infection seen.

Median survival 40 years.

Investigations: Sweat test, genetic screening.

Treatment: Chest physiotherapy, bronchodilators, i.v. antibiotics for exacerbations, DNA'ase, pancreatic enzyme supplements.

Patients suffering from CF can develop bronchiectasis.

Trigger box   Bronchiectasis

Permanent bronchial dilatation.

CF most common cause, also idiopathic, postinfective (measles, pneumonia, pertussis), cilial disorders.

Findings: Cough, sputum, haemoptysis, clubbing, crackles, wheezing.

Investigations: High resolution CT, sputum culture.

Treatment: Physiotherapy, antibiotics, bronchodilators, steroids.

Table 1.6 Age of patient and the pathogens causing pneumonia

Age	Pathogens
Neonates	Group B streptococcus, *E. coli.*
Children	Respiratory syncytial virus, *Mycoplasma pneumoniae,* *Chlamydia pneumoniae, Streptococcus pneumoniae*
Young adults	*Mycoplasma pneumoniae*
Older adults & elderly	*Streptococcus pneumoniae*

Irene's chest X-ray showed left lower lobe consolidation suggesting lobar pneumonia. This was confirmed by the sputum culture, which revealed *Streptococcus pneumoniae*. So, Irene was suffering from a chest infection with underlying COPD.

People like Irene who suffer from COPD also suffer from frequent pulmonary infections like pneumonia. The pathogens causing pneumonia depend on the age of the patient, as shown in Table 1.6.

Trigger box   Pneumonia

Inflammation of lung tissue.

Findings: Pyrexia, cough, sputum, pleurisy, dyspnoea, consolidation, pleural rub, pleural effusion, confusion (elderly).

Blood cultures positive in 20% cases even if sputum is negative: indicates poor prognosis.

Risk factors: Smoking, alcoholism, lung disease, immunosuppression, chronic disease.

Investigations: CXR, FBC (WBC $> 15 \times 10^9$/L suggests bacterial infection), cold agglutinins in *Mycoplasma pneumoniae*, raised urea and hypoalbunimia = severe pneumonia, arterial blood gases (ABG) (PaO_2 <8 kPa/hypercarbia = severe pneumonia).

Main pathogens

1. Community acquired: *Streptococcus pneumoniae* (70%). *Mycoplasma pneumoniae.* (15%), *Chlamydia* spp. (7%).
2. Hospital acquired: Gram-negative bacteria (50%).

Treatment:

Community acquired – amoxicillin.

Penicillin allergics – erythromycin or azithromycin.

Staphylococcus aureus – flucloxacillin.

Physiotherapy.

Complications: Lung abscess, empyema.

Mortality 25% in elderly.

Irene has chronic bronchitis, her brother Ted has emphysema. These diseases are part of a group of conditions (together with chronic asthma) that make up COPD. Most COPD sufferers are smokers.

Trigger box   COPD

Decreased FEV_1; decreased FEV_1/FVC; increased TLC; increased RV.
Chronic bronchitis/emphysema.
Most are smokers.

Chronic bronchitis (blue bloater):
Features: Productive cough >3/12 for 2 consecutive years, hypercarbia, hypoxia, hyper inflated lungs.

Emphysema (pink puffer):
Centriolobular (smoking); panlobular (α_1 antitrypsin deficiency).
Features: Dyspnoea, decreased breath sounds, hypercarbia, hypoxia, bullae.

Treatment: O_2, beta agonists, ipratropium, steroids, antibiotics.

Can you describe the significance of α_1-antitrypsin to emphysema?

Smokers are also at a high risk of developing lung cancer. Study the Trigger Box on lung cancer.

Trigger box   Lung cancer

Most common malignant tumour.
Types:

1. *Non small cell* (70–80%)

   Squamous cell carcinoma (40%), large cell carcinoma (25%) adenocarcinoma (10%).

2. *Small cell* (20–30%).

Causes: Smoking, asbestos.
Features: Cough, chest pain, hemoptysis, finger clubbing, Pancoast's tumour, Horner's syndrome, superior vena cava (SVC) obstruction.

Investigations: CXR, sputum cytology, bronchoscopy, CT, MRI (for Pancoast's tumour)
Treatment: Non small cell – surgery, radiotherapy or chemotherapy. Small cell – chemotherapy $\pm$ radiotherapy.

Irene could develop cyanosis and become a 'blue bloater'. Ted uses his accessory muscles and gets exhausted. He is thin, has a barrel chest and his lungs are fast losing their elasticity and shows high compliance. He has heard Dr Blunt referring to him as a pink puffer.

Let us return to Irene in hospital. The doctor sat next to her and began advising her against smoking when Irene interrupted him politely. She had given up smoking.

'I know all about how bad smoking can be,' said Irene. 'I know . . . look what it did to poor Ted. He's got emphysema you know'.

Patients with COPD without hypercarbia can be treated with 100 per cent O_2 through a facemask. This improves alveolar ventilation. Since the ventilation/perfusion ratio has to be matched arterioles supplying these alveoli dilate so as to increase perfusion. For gas exchange to be efficient there must be match between ventilation and perfusion. You need to know about ventilation and perfusion (Figure 1.8).

Trigger box   **Pulmonary embolism (PE)**

Usually due to a deep venous thrombosis (DVT); how does a DVT cause a PE?
V/Q mismatch
Findings: dyspnoea, pleuritic chest pain, haemoptysis, or if severe shock, syncope and death.
Central cyanosis, elevated JVP (jugular venous pressure), right ventricular (RV) heave, loud heart sound (HS) 2, gallop rhythm
Investigations: VQ scan, D dimers, Doppler US, CT, pulmonary angiogram
Treatment: Oxygen, streptokinase, morphine, i.v. heparin/warfarin for prevention, i.v. fluids, inotropes, vena caval filter.

What is the key difference between systemic capillaries and pulmonary capillaries in terms of their response when flowing through hypoxic regions?

Uncle Ted came to visit Irene in hospital. He looked a bit perturbed. He mentioned a conversation he had overheard between Dr Blunt and a medical student, where his increased dead space had been discussed. Dead space refers to the volume that is ventilated but does not participate in gas exchange. Anatomical dead space includes all the conduit airways down to bronchioles. Since Ted has air in his conduction system

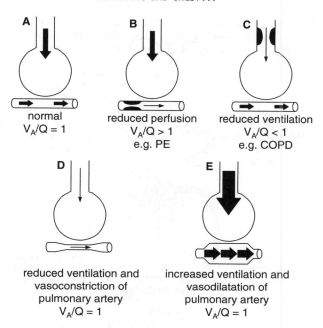

Figure 1.8 Ventilation and perfusion. 'D' and 'E' shows how vasodilatation or vasoconstriction corrects a V_A/Q mismatch

The V/Q ratio $=$ alveolar ventilation rate/pulmonary blood flow
If there is no ventilation, $Va/Q = 0$
For example you get perfusion without ventilation when an alveolus is full of liquid as in severe pneumonia. This will reduce arterial PaO_2.
If there is no perfusion, $Va/Q = \infty$
Here the alveoli are ventilated but not perfused, for example due to a pulmonary embolus.
Remember pulmonary vessels constrict in poorly ventilated regions.
A pulmonary embolus is a medical emergency and causes a severe V/Q mismatch.

and lots of destroyed alveoli, which do not participate in gas exchange, he has lots of dead space! Physiological dead space includes alveoli that are ventilated but not perfused, which occurs in patients suffering with pulmonary emboli.

Note: alveolar ventilation rate $=$ (tidal vol – dead space) $\times$ respiratory rate

 Dead space is increased in artificial respiration when the patient is connected to tubing. What physiological effects will this have on the patient's tidal volume and respiratory rate?

After talking about dead space, Dr Blunt had gone on to describe things that caused Ted to experience even more fear.

'The loss of functional alveoli in emphysema,' he had said, 'will reduce diffusion capacity and therefore impair gas exchange. You can also see this in pulmonary oedema.'

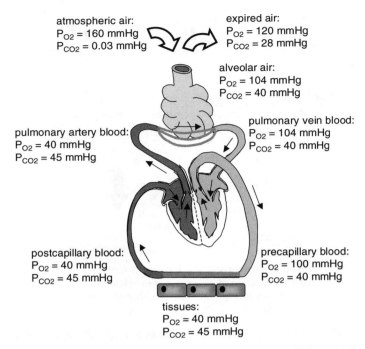

atmospheric air:
P_{O2} = 160 mmHg
P_{CO2} = 0.03 mmHg

expired air:
P_{O2} = 120 mmHg
P_{CO2} = 28 mmHg

alveolar air:
P_{O2} = 104 mmHg
P_{CO2} = 40 mmHg

pulmonary artery blood:
P_{O2} = 40 mmHg
P_{CO2} = 45 mmHg

pulmonary vein blood:
P_{O2} = 104 mmHg
P_{CO2} = 40 mmHg

postcapillary blood:
P_{O2} = 40 mmHg
P_{CO2} = 45 mmHg

precapillary blood:
P_{O2} = 100 mmHg
P_{CO2} = 40 mmHg

tissues:
P_{O2} = 40 mmHg
P_{CO2} = 45 mmHg

Figure 1.9   Gas exchange. Adapted from Sherwood (2004) Human Physiology from Cells to System, 5th edition, Thomson, Brooks/Cole.

Figure 1.9 shows changes in PaO_2 and $PaCO_2$ as blood moves from metabolically active tissues to the lungs and back.

What drives the movement of these gases from tissue to venous blood, from venous blood to alveoli, from alveoli to arterial blood and from arterial blood to tissue?
Why is PaO_2 in systemic arterial blood lower than that in pulmonary veins?
Which hormone increases RBC formation? Where is it produced?

List the causes of pulmonary oedema.

How is diffusion capacity measured?
What conditions reduce diffusion capacity?

Zoe's oxygen saturation at the height of her asthma attack was 78 per cent. After treatment it rose to 98 per cent. You need to know about haemoglobin (Hb) and O_2 saturation curves. O_2 carrying capacity of the blood is proportional to the Hb concentration in the alveoli. Hb has four O_2 binding sites. The shape of the dissociation curve is

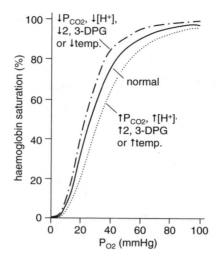

Figure 1.10 Oxygen dissociation curves (also shows the Bohr effect). Adapted from McGeown (1999) Physiology, Churchill Livingstone

due to the fact that binding of one Hb molecule increases the binding capacity of other sites. Factors, which shift the O_2 dissociation curve, are shown in Figure 1.10.

The physiological significance of these shifts is seen when it is appreciated that all factors that shift the curve to the right are seen in systemic capillaries where O_2 unloading is the goal.

 Can you explain the significance of increased 2-3 diphosphoglycerate (DPG)?

The Bohr effect is seen when the $PaCO_2$ levels are increased. The curve shifts to the right so that the O_2 saturation is lower for a given PaO_2. Hence the curve for systemic venous blood with higher $PaCO_2$ lies to the right of arterial blood. This increases O_2 extraction as blood flows through actively respiring tissues that generate CO_2.

Different types of Hb also affect O_2 dissociation curves. Figure 1.11 shows O_2 dissociation curves for fetal Hb and myoglobin.

 Describe the significance of the shapes of the dissociation curves of fetal haemoglobin and myoglobin.

Some conditions reduce O_2 affinity of haemoglobin. Example when Fe^{2+} is converted Fe^{3+} to form methaemoglobin which has a reduced O_2 binding capacity.

 List the main causes of methaemaglobinaemia.

A few years ago there was a fire two houses down from the Sikalott home. Fortunately no one died but several people had to be taken to hospital with carbon monoxide

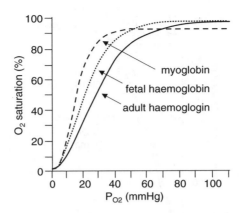

Figure 1.11   Dissociation curves for different oxygen carriers. Adapted from McGeown (1999) Physiology, Churchill Livingstone

poisoning. CO binds with greater affinity to haemoglobin than O_2 and forms carboxyhemoglobin, as seen in Figure 1.12.

?   *Why do patients suffering from CO poisoning appear a pink - red colour?*

Let us now consider CO_2 transport.
   CO_2 is transported in three forms:

1. As HCO_3 (60–70 per cent). (See Figure 1.13)

2. In carbamino groups - mostly binding to Hb (20–30 per cent).

3. As dissolved gas (10 per cent).

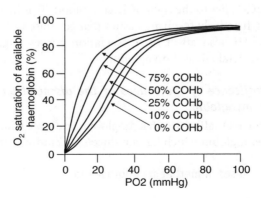

Figure 1.12   The effects of carbon monoxide on the oxygen carrying capacity of blood. Adapted from www.coheadquarters.com/cohaldane1.htm

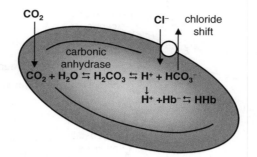

Figure 1.13 Carbon dioxide metabolism in the erythrocyte. Adapted from Ganong (1991) Review of Medical Physiology, 15th edition, Appleton & Lange

What is the chloride shift

CO_2 dissociation curves (not shown) show higher CO_2 concentrations at a given $PaCO_2$ when compared to the situation in the O_2 dissociation curve. This is because CO_2 is more soluble. Also when comparing to the O_2 dissociation curve, CO_2 has a narrower physiological range and no plateau.

The Haldane effect describes how the CO_2 dissociation curve shifts down and to the left when the PaO_2 is increased. Hence the CO_2 concentration drops at a given $PaCO_2$. The Haldane effect increases the uptake of CO_2 from respiring tissues. The Haldane effect is due to deoxygenated Hb being able to carry more CO_2 in the carbamino form and because it is a more effective pH buffer than oxyhaemoglobin. The Haldane effect is shown in Figure 1.14.

Whilst in hospital Ted found out that someone in the next room was having an even tougher time. He overheard Dr Blunt explaining- to his student – that "this fellow was

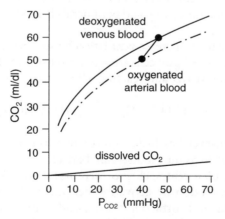

Figure 1.14 The Haldane effect. Adapted from McGeown (1999) Physiology, Churchill Livingstone

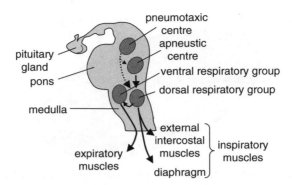

Figure 1.15 Respiratory centres showing stimulatory (solid arrows) and inhibitory (dotted arrows) pathway connections. Adapted from Tortora and Grabowski (2003), Principles of Antomy and Physiology, 10th edition, John Wiley & Sons

showing apneustic breathing – long inspiratory breaths followed by brief exhalations". Dr Blunt explained that "breathing was regulated by the brain stem" and that "this fellow had had a stroke that had caused damage to his pons" – whatever that is! This brings us to the control of respiration, which is shown, in Figure 1.15.

Inspiratory respiratory neurones in the medulla (DRG) stimulate motor neurones reaching the diaphragm and external intercostals. These inspiratory respiratory neurones show spontaneous rhythmical activity with pauses, which cause expiration to occur passively.

Expiratory respiratory neurons (VRG) only become active during episodes of increased (forced) ventilation. These stimulate motor neurons causing internal intercostals and abdominal muscles to contract. Respiratory cells in the pons are not essential for respiration but can modify the pattern of breathing. The pontine pneumotaxic centre inhibits inspiratory neurons and shortens inspiration.

You need to understand the central and peripheral chemoreceptor control of respiration shown in Figure 1.16.

Increases in arterial PaCO$_2$ increase ventilation by stimulating central chemoreceptors in the medulla. Chemoreceptor cells are actually sensitive to H$^+$ ions formed by CO$_2$ crossing the blood–brain barrier and reacting with water:

$$CO_2 + H_2O \leftrightharpoons H_2CO_3 \leftrightharpoons H^+ + HCO_3^-$$

An arterial acidosis however has little immediate effect on central chemoreceptors because H$^+$ ions cannot cross the blood–brain barrier.

In contrast PaO$_2$ stimulate central chemoreceptors less well. However if PaO$_2$ drops a lot it can stimulate ventilation by activating peripheral chemoreceptors. Peripheral chemoreceptors (carotid and aortic bodies) respond to increased arterial pH and low PaO$_2$. Hypoxia of an adequate degree will therefore stimulate ventilation via peripheral chemoreceptors.

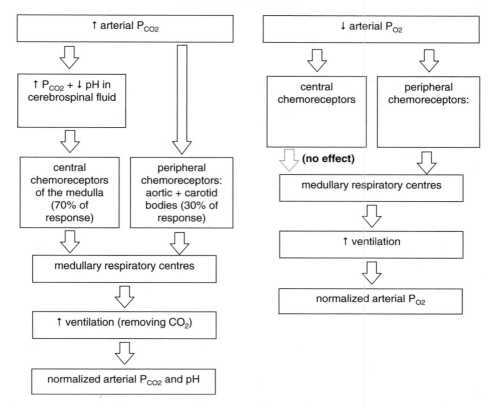

Figure 1.16 Central and peripheral chemoreceptor control of breathing

Irene has hypoxic drive because her $PaCO_2$ is chronically elevated due to her COPD. Her central chemoreceptors have become unresponsive and her oxygen sensitive peripheral chemoreceptors now respond to lowered PaO_2.

You have to be careful giving her 100 per cent O_2 because this can remove the stimulus for her breathing.

What happens if the spinal cord in transected just below the pons?

Describe the main changes seen in respiratory physiology in (a) high altitude, (b) vigorous exercise

2

The cardiovascular system

Learning strategy

In this chapter we will consider the essential, 'must know' facts and concepts of the cardiovascular system. Our main strategy will involve an exploration of these key principles by following several clinical scenarios.

An angina scenario will lead us to consider the structure and embryology of the heart. A cardiovascular physical examination will lead us to look at cardiac function. This will include consideration of valve function and disorders. Blood loss caused by a stabbing will allow us to consider the concept of cardiac output. COPD leading to right heart failure (RHF) will lead us to an exploration of heart failure. Returning to the angina patient we will go on to consider blood pressure physiology, hypertension and hyperlipidemia focussing on their mechanisms and treatment strategies.

An acute myocardial infarction (MI) scenario will lead to a consideration of the pathophysiology and treatment of MI and cardiac arrhythmia.

Throughout, we will also consider the pathophysiological mechanisms of several key conditions and disease states involving the cardiovascular system, which will, in addition to highlighting the key pathophysiological principles, further reinforce basic principles of anatomy, physiology and pharmacology relevant to the system.

Try to answer the questions and carry out the Learning task. Use the Trigger boxes for rapid revision of key facts.

John is a worried man . . .

It was spring. The long, cold wet winter had finally come to an end. But the warmer weather, blooming flowers or the happy sounds of spring did not bring any joy to John.

Integrated Medical Sciences   by Shantha Perera, Stephen Anderson, Ho Leung and Rousseau Gama
© 2007 John Wiley & Sons, Ltd   ISBN: 978470016589 (HB) 978470016596 (PB)

He was definitely under the weather. Something was wrong, but John couldn't quite put his finger on it. He felt run down, lacked energy and even lost interest in his usual pleasures like visiting the pub every evening or football on Saturday. In fact he had even gone off his cigarettes and his beer!

He had two, more tangible problems. The first was the calf pain that came on whenever he walked for about 50 metres. The second, and more worrying, was a dull chest pain that also came on occasionally when he exerted himself. Both problems made their appearance more often when John climbed Sunnybrook Hill, a short cut to his house from the bus stop. He also became breathless when walking uphill. The pain went away once he rested, but his feet felt cold most of the time. Once recently the chest pains had come on when he was making love. Mary was not amused!

What concerned John, who was 51, was the knowledge that his dad had died of a heart attack at 60 and that his brother, Dick, was born with a hole in the heart and had to have an operation when he was just a few months old.

'Maybe, the hearts in our family aren't put together properly', John used to say and claimed that his problems were all 'genetic'. 'It doesn't matter if I eat 10 burgers a day or drink 10 pints, in the end my ticker will pack up. We have lousy hearts in our family.'

We will begin our exploration of the cardiovascular system by considering its development. The cardiovascular system is mesodermal in origin. The main embryological developmental stages of the heart are shown in Figure 2.1.

So, when do the key events occur? By day 22 the heart tube is formed. During 4th to 7th week the heart has its four chambers. The heart begins to beat by week 4.

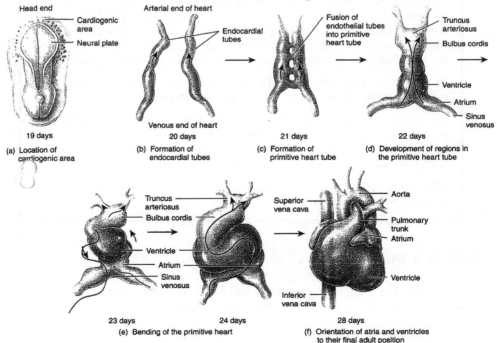

Figure 2.1 Development of the heart. Adapted from Tortora and Grabowski (2003), Principles of Anatomy and Physiology, 10th Edition, John Wiley and Sons Inc. New York

Table 2.1 Common congenital cardiac defects

Early cyanotic

R to L shunts.
Tetralogy of Fallot
Transposition of great vessels
Truncus arteriosus
(Note: All start with a T)

Late cyanotic

L to R shunts
Ventricular septal defect (VSD) (Most common)
Atrial septal defect (ASD)
Patent ductus arteriosus (PDA)
(Note: All have a D)

 List the derivatives of the aortic arches.

Septum formation is partly due to the development of an endocardial cushion in the AV canal and in the truncoconal regions. Many congenital cardiac abnormalities are related to cushion malformations. Common congenital cardiac defects are listed in Table 2.1 John's brother Dick had a ventricular septal defect (VSD).

 Find out the key features of these conditions. How and when are they treated?

Figure 2.2 shows the some of the more common congenital heart defects. For simplicity these are all indicated in a single heart. It is important to understand the significance of Right to Left and Left to Right shunting.

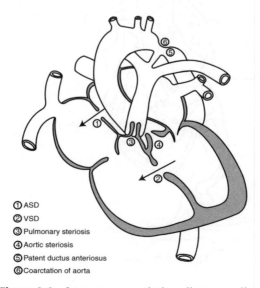

① ASD
② VSD
③ Pulmonary steriosis
④ Aortic steriosis
⑤ Patent ductus anteriosus
⑥ Coarctation of aorta

Figure 2.2 Common congenital cardiac anomalies.

Which four anomalies constitute the tetralogy of Fallot?
Uncorrected VSD, ASD, or PDA can lead to progressive pulmonary hypertension.
Why?
Shunt changes to L to R causes late cyanosis. Why?
What is Eisenmenger's syndrome?

Figures 2.3 and 2.4 show foetal and neonatal circulations.

Note that in the foetus the umbilical vein carries oxygenated blood to the heart. Blood coming via the IVC is mainly diverted through the foramen ovale and pumped out of the aorta to the head. Deoxygenated blood coming from the SVC is mainly expelled into the pulmonary artery and via the ductus arteriosus supply the lower body. This arrangement ensures that the developing brain gets the best blood! At birth, the first breath decreases pulmonary resistance causing increased left atrial pressure causing the foramen ovale to close. Eventually the ductus arteriosus also closes.

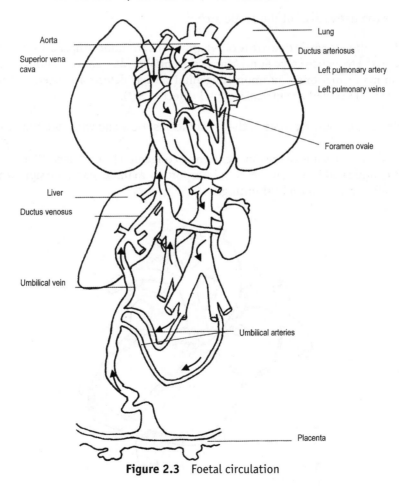

Figure 2.3 Foetal circulation

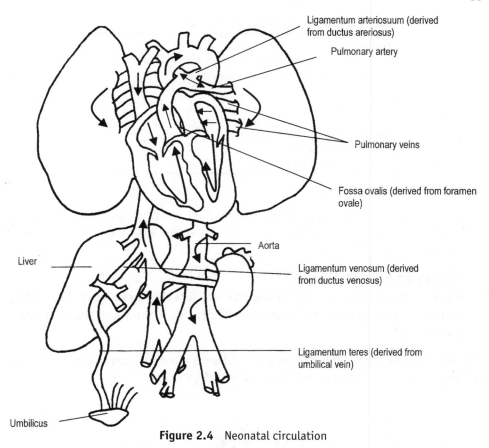

Figure 2.4 Neonatal circulation

What are the functions of the foramen ovale and ductus arteriosus?
What congenital conditions require a patent ductus for survival?
How is patent ductus treated?
What are the signs of coarctation of the aorta?

The interruption to their lovemaking, which was getting pretty infrequent of late anyway, was the last straw for Mary. She insisted on John visiting Dr Smith.

Dr Smith wasn't in the best of moods. John wasn't a model patient; and turning up 20 minutes late for his appointment, didn't help. He had also failed to attend his two last hypertension clinics. John mentioned his chest pains and asked for some medicine.

Dr Smith carried out a quick history, which revealed a classic angina type of pain. He also noted that John had several risk factors for heart disease.

The modifiable non-modifiable risk factors for cardiovascular disease are shown in Table 2.2 below.

Table 2.2 Major cardiovascular risk factors

Male gender.
Family history of premature coronary artery disease (CAD).
Ethnicity – Indoasians >Caucasians.
Increasing age.
Hypertension.
Smoking.
Diabetes mellitus (types 1 and 2)
High LDL cholesterol.
Low HDL cholesterol.

Dr Smith then began his examination. John showed a normal apex beat and normal heart sounds 1 and 2. There were no murmurs. His pulse was 90 and regular and his blood pressure was 150/97.

Is John's BP normal?
Where did Dr Smith place the stethoscope to ausculate the four valves of the heart?
What causes the normal heart sounds? What does a third and fourth heart sound signify?

The praecordial examination leads us to consider the gross anatomy of the heart, which is shown in Figure 2.5. Figure 2.6 shows the histology of heart tissue.

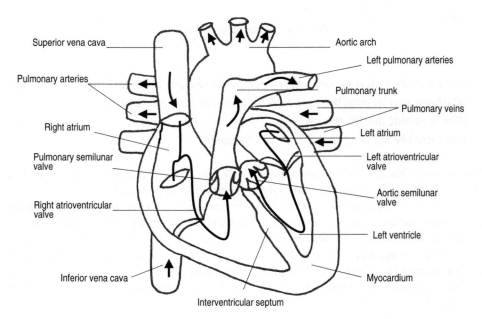

Figure 2.5 Anatomy of the heart

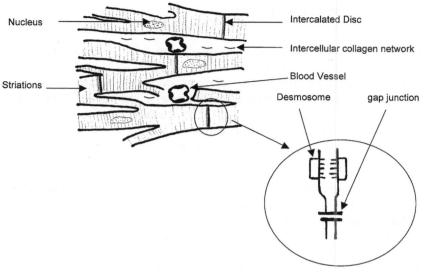

Figure 2.6 Cardiac muscle histology

Compare and contrast the histology of cardiac muscle with that of smooth and striated muscle

What is the function of cardiac gap junctions?

The heart is covered by the thin pericardium, inflammation of which leads to the important condition pericarditis.

Trigger box **Pericarditis**

Acute inflammation of pericardium
Causes: Infection (e.g. Coxsackie virus), myocardial infarction, connective tissue disease (e.g. systemic lupus erythematosus), neoplasms, drugs, metabolic (uraemia).
Features: Sharp chest pain relieved by leaning forward; worse on inspiration; pericardial friction rub, upsloping ST elevation except in AVR and V1.
Complications: Pericardial effusion and tamponade. Pleural fluid on Echocardiogram.
Treatment: Treat underlying disease, NSAIDs, steroids.
Aspirate tamponade.

If Dr Smith had heard a *murmur* that would have indicated a valve disorder, which could have been confirmed by echocardiography.

Trigger Box: Common valve disorders

1. *Aortic stenosis*
Causes: Calcification of normal valve, rheumatic fever (RF), congenital malformation
Results in left ventricular hypertrophy (LVH).
Features: Often asymptomatic, exertional dyspnoea, syncope, angina.
Physical examination: Plateau pulse, LVH (sustained and heaving apex beat), aortic
ejection mid systolic murmur radiating into the carotids.
Complications: Left ventricular failure, endocarditis.
Treatment: valve replacement if symptomatic or severe stenosis.

2. *Aortic regurgitation*
Causes: Congenital malformation, endocarditis, RF, connective tissue diseases.
Features: Asymptomatic, dyspnoea, less often, angina.
Physical examination: Wide pulse pressure (collapsing pulse); LVH (sustained and
heaving apex beat), early aortic diastolic murmur, Austin Flint murmur (apical systolic
murmur).
Complications: Left ventricular failure, endocarditis.
Treatment: treat heart failure (diuretics), valve replacement.

3. *Mitral stenosis*
Causes: Due to rheumatic fever.
Results in low cardiac output; increased pulmonary arterial pressure, right ventricular
hypertrophy (RVH).
Features: Worsening dyspnoea, palpitations (atrial fibrillation), emboli, haemoptysis.
Physical examination: Irregularly irregular pulse (atrial fibrillation), RVH (left para-
sternal heave), loud HS1, opening snap, mid-diastolic murmur.
Complications: Right ventricular failure, AF, emboli, endocarditis.
Treatment: Treat AF with digitalis, beta blockers, anticoagulation to prevent emboli,
diuretics for heart failure, balloon vulvoplasty, valve replacement.

4. *Mitral regurgitation*
Causes: Most common cause is mitral prolapse. Other causes include endocarditis, RF,
myocardial infarction, left ventricular dilatation.
Features: Worsening dyspnoea.
Physical examination: AF, LVH, apical pansystolic murmur.
Complications: Left ventricular failure, less often AF, emboli, endocarditis.
Treatment: Treat heart failure with diuretics, angiotensin-converting enzyme inhibitor
(ACEI), valvuloplasty or valve replacement.

By considering *how* the valve normally functions, try to figure out *why* the murmur is
systolic or diastolic. For example, when the heart is in systole blood goes through the
aortic valve. If this is stenosed you hear the murmur, which is systolic!!
    Heart valves can get infected, a condition called bacterial endocarditis

---

Trigger box **Bacterial endocarditis**

Infection of endocardium/vascular endothelium.

Generally subacute.

Valves with congenital or acquired defects, normal and prosthetics all affected.

Right sided endocarditis – intravenous drug abuse (IVDA).

Most common (50%) *Streptococcus mutans*, *Streptococcus sanguis* (why?), *Staphylococcus aureus* in IVDA.

Vegetations can cause regurgitation, congestive heart failure (CHF).

Features: Malaise, fever, anemia, changing murmurs, emboli and metastatic abscesses, immune complex deposition; vasculitis, splinter haemorrhages, Osler nodes, Roth's spots, Janeway lesions, arthralgia, glomerulonephritis.

Investigations: Blood cultures, ECHO to see vegetations.

Treatment: Empirical: benzyl penicillin and gentamicin.

Prevention: At risk prophylactic antibiotics eg dental work.

? *What is the aetiology of rheumatic fever? What are its signs and symptoms? Arial myxomas can cause valve blockage. What are the features of atrial myxoma?*

'How's my pulse, Doc?' John asked.

'It's a little high, but it's regular' Dr Smith replied. John already knew that his pulse was regular. He was checking his pulse often and was amazed at its regularity.

'What makes my heartbeat regular, Doc?' he asked. Dr Smith explained that the pacemaker of the heart was responsible for the regular beat. Cardiac action potentials, the pacemaker potential and conduction pathways are shown in Figures 2.7, 2.8 and 2.9.

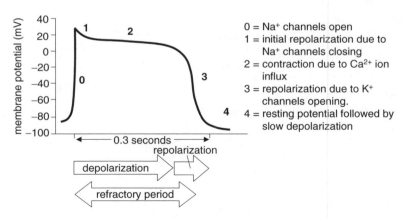

0 = Na⁺ channels open
1 = initial repolarization due to Na⁺ channels closing
2 = contraction due to Ca^{2+} ion influx
3 = repolarization due to K⁺ channels opening.
4 = resting potential followed by slow depolarization

Figure 2.7 Cardiac action potential. Adapted from Tortora and Grabowski (2003), Principles of Anatomy and Physiology, 10th edition, John Wiley & Sons

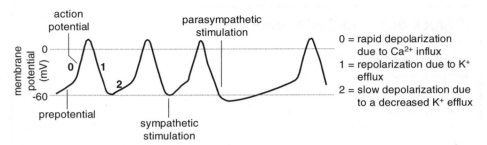

Figure 2.8 Pacemaker potential showing the effects of sympathetic and parasympathetic stimulation on prepotentials. Adapted from Rang, Dale, Ritter and Moore, (2003) Pharmacology, 5th edition, Churchill Livingstone

Abnormalities involving the electrical activity of the heart give rise to conduction defects.

Trigger box   Conduction abnormalities

First degree heart block
Prolonged PR interval (>0.2 s).
No treatment required.

Second degree heart block
1. Mobitz type 1 (Wenkebach): PR gradually increases then absent QRS.

Observation.
2. Mobitz type 2: dropped QRS *not* preceded by progressive prolonged PR.

3. 2:1 or 3:1 block: QRS after every second/third P conduction.

Pacing required.

Third degree heart block
No association between P and QRS.
Dizziness, blackouts (Stokes Adams attacks).
Permanent pacemaker required.

Intraventricular conduction defects
Increased QRS duration.
Often asymptomatic, no treatment required unless post MI.

1. RBBB: rSR with wide R in V1: QRS with wide S in V6.

2. LBBB: Wide negative QS in V1: Wide R without Q in V6.

LBBB, left bundle branch block; RBBB, right bundle branch block.

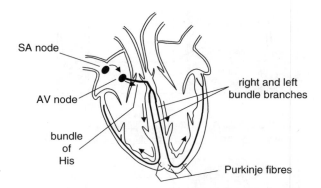

Figure 2.9 Cardiac conduction pathway. Arrows indicate direction of action potentials

What is Wolf–Parkinson–White syndrome? How is it treated?

Dr Smith next asked the Practice Nurse to carry out an ECG, which showed a normal sinus rhythm, but with evidence of left ventricular hypertrophy, and one premature ventricular beat.

What is the significance of the left ventricular hypertrophy? What is the most likely mechanism causing LVH?

The normal ECG is shown in Figure 2.10. Note the atrial and ventricular depolarizations that result in contraction.

What are the typical ECG changes in hyperkalaemia?

We can now consider the stages of the cardiac cycle, which is shown in Figure 2.11. Note how the ECG stages relate to the other parameters.

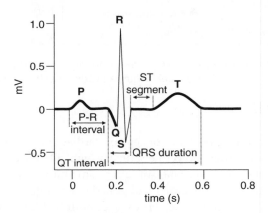

Figure 2.10 The normal ECG

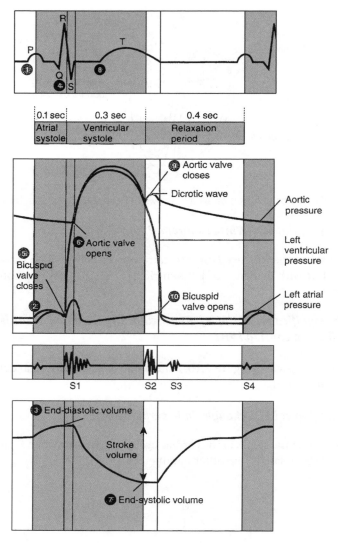

Figure 2.11 The Cardiac cycle. Adapted from Tortora and Grabowski (2003), Principles of Anatomy and Physiology, 10th Edition, John Wiley and Sons Inc. New York

Max is attacked!

We can next look at the important concept of cardiac output by considering what happened to Debbie's boyfriend Max one Saturday night. On the night in question, Max had been visited by a drug dealer who was after some money owed to him. Max had started arguing with him and the dealer had pulled out a knife and stabbed Max in the abdomen. Luckily, a few minutes later Max's neighbour had found him on the landing lying in a pool of blood. She had immediately called the ambulance.

Max was rushed into the Emergency Department(ED) at Hope Hospital.

'He's tachycardic,' the paramedic reported as Max was wheeled into a cubicle. 'Pulse 112, BP 70/25.'

What does the high heart rate and low BP signify?

'Let's start an IV,' the emergency doctor said. 'Push some fluids in and cross match two units. We don't want his cardiac output to drop any more'.

The different types of fluids given under different conditions are shown in Table 2.3.

Table 2.3 Intravenous fluids

Crystalloid solutions

True solution.

Stays in the intravascular compartment for short period (compared to colloids).

Useful to replace volume rapidly after sudden blood loss (with colloids), replacing GI losses from NG suction, and vomiting. Postoperative treatment.

Examples: Na lactate, NaCl 0.9% (normal saline), NaCl 0.18% + glucose 4% (normovolaemic, normonatraemic patients), glucose 5% + KCl 0.3% + sodium bicarbonate 1.26% (volume expansion in hypovolaemic, acidotic patients).

Colloids

Do not dissolve into true solution.

Stays in the intravascular compartment for longer (compared to crystalloid). Increases oncotic pressure.

Useful to replace volume rapidly after sudden blood loss (with crystalloid).

Interfere with cross matching, allergic reactions.

Examples; dextran, haemacel, gelofusin, hydroxyethyl starches.

Blood products

Packed red cells; use in major bleeding or severe acute anaemia. Can use O negative in emergency.Whole blood is used rarely.

Human albumin solutions: used to correct a plasma-volume deficit in patients with salt and water retention and oedema (e.g. burns and peritonitis) where there is loss of plasma protein, water and electrolytes. Also used to achieve diuresis in hypoalbuminaemic patients (e.g. in hepatic cirrhosis) but not appropriate for treating hypoalbuminaemia only.

Fresh frozen plasma: coagulation defects. *Not* a plasma expander. Monitor with PT test.

Platelets: severe thrombocytopenia.

Acute bleed: What to do

Stem any external bleeding.

Insert a wide-bore cannula.

Take blood for cross matching.

Rapid infusion of normal saline followed by colloid.

Give blood as soon as it becomes available (cross matched).

NB: If you under correct fluid loss patient could develop renal failure.
If you overcorrect patient could develop pulmonary oedema and heart failure.

Max survived.

'Your cardiac output was falling,' the doctor who treated him told him later. 'That is why your heart was racing. When we pushed the fluids in, the cardiac output increased.'

Stab wounds to the chest can cause tamponade. What is tamponade and how is it treated?

Max has often used cocaine. What are the cardiovascular effects of cocaine? What are the mechanisms involved?

Cardiac output is an important concept you really must understand. It is the product of heart rate (HR) and stroke volume (SV) which is the volume of blood ejected from the left ventricle during one contraction. The formula and method of measurement of CO is as follows:

$$CO = HR \times SV$$

So for a heart rate of 80 bpm and a stroke volume of 60 ml (0.06 L) the cardiac output would be $4.8 \, L \, min^{-1}$.

Fick's equation can be used to measure CO using the following formula:

CO = rate of oxygen consumption/arterial oxygen concentration – venous

oxygen concentration.

So which factors affect the cardiac ouput? Heart rate is affected by the activity of the autonomic nervous system (increased by the SNS and decreased by the PNS). Heart rate is also increased by adrenaline, noradrenaline and thyroid hormones. *Chronotrophs* increase heart rate.

Stroke volume is regulated by contractility, preload and afterload. Contractility is the strength of contraction at any given preload and afterload. *Positive inotrophs* increase contractility whereas *negative inotrophs* decrease contractility.

Let us now focus on the important concepts of *preload* and *afterload*. *Preload* is the amount of stretch experienced by relaxed cardiac muscle cells just before contraction. Increasing venous return increases this stretch by increasing *end diastolic volume* and pressure which causes an increased force of contraction and so more blood is ejected from the heart.

The end diastolic volume is the volume of blood contained in the ventricles by the end of ventricular diastole. The length of resting cardiac muscle fibres is determined by venous filling and is normally less than the optimal length necessary for generating maximum tension. Increasing venous return increase end diastolic volume, which stretches muscle fibres closer to their optimal lengths and increases the force of contraction for the next systole.

Afterload is the pressure that has to be exceeded for blood to be ejected from the ventricles and is caused by arterial blood exerting back pressure on the semilunar valves. Afterload equals the amount of resistance to blood flow into the aorta and peripheral arteries (total peripheral resistance).

The Frank–Starling curve is the representation of ventricular function obtained by constructing a graph of mean left atrial pressure or end diastolic pressure or volume

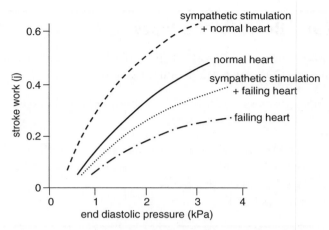

Figure 2.12   Frank–Starling curve shifts. Adapted from Boron and Boulpaep (2003), Medical Physiology, Suanders

against either cardiac output or stroke volume or stroke work. Such a graph demonstrates that increasing venous return or mean left atrial pressure increases cardiac output until the point where the heart becomes overloaded and output begins to fall.

When Max was infused with saline it restored the volume in the vasculature. This in turn increased the amount of blood filling the ventricles, the preload. This then caused an increase in the cardiac output in accordance with Starling's Law (Figure 2.12). The heart, not needing to beat as fast to maintain cardiac output, started to slow down.

More problems for Irene...

Meanwhile, down the road, in the bungalow, Irene was developing her own set of problems, which necessitated another visit to see Dr Smith.

She was becoming more fatigued, and, like John, also became short of breath with exertion. Worryingly, she found even climbing the stairs very difficult.

Dr Smith examined her. He found poor chest expansion and laboured respiratory effort with intercostal indrawing on inspration and pursing of lips on expiration. He also detected hyperresonance to percussion, diminished breath sounds, wheezing and distant heart sounds. She also had a raised JVP and her feet were swollen.

What is the significance of these clinical findings?
What does the increased JVP signify?

He was concerned that Irene, with her long term COPD was developing right-sided heart failure. Was her fatigue reflecting a relative inability to increase cardiac output during exertion? He decided to refer her to Dr Hart, the consultant cardiologist at Hope Hospital.

Trigger box   Heart failure types

1. *Systolic failure* (forward failure) = Left ventricle (LV) fails to eject blood. Cardiac output (CO) may fall and reduce tissue perfusion.

2. *Diastolic failure* (backward failure) = LV cannot relax in diastole so cannot fill adequately.

Left heart failure (LHF) causes pulmonary congestion and pleural effusions.
Right heart failure (RHF) causes increased JVP, hepatic congestion (hepatomegaly), peripheral (sacral and leg) oedema and ascites.
The main cause of RHF is LHF!!

Irene's feet were swollen. Describe the mechanisms of oedema formation in CHF. What are Starling's forces and how do they interact to cause oedema?

Dr Smith asked Irene how many pillows she used at night and if she had to periodically get up and walk about during the night because of shortness of breath. What is the significance of these questions?
Why are dobutamine and dopamine sometimes used in the treatment of CHF?
What is the role of beta blockers and ACE inhibitors in the treatment of CHF?

Another important disease state that is relevant to our consideration of heart failure is cardiomyopathy, which can present with CHF.
Irene attended Hope hospital. Dr Hart confirmed the raised JVP, an enlarged tender liver and ankle oedema consistent with RHF.

A right-sided fourth heart sound was also present and reflected the increase in the filling pressure of the right ventricle. The chest X-ray showed enlargement of the central pulmonary arteries. The X-ray also showed an increase of the transverse diameter of the heart.

What radiological feature indicated an enlarged heart?
Can you explain the mechanisms underlying these clinical findings?

'We need to check her ejection fraction,' he said to a nurse. 'Let's do an echo'.

Which disease states are monitored by echocardiography?

The concept of ejection fraction is shown below:
E_f = (End diastolic volume – End systolic volume)/End Diastolic volume
   = Stroke Volume (SV)/End diastolic volume
   = 60–70%
Irene's ejection fraction was found to be 40 per cent.

Trigger box Cardiomyopathy

Types:

1. *Dilated cardiomyopathy*
   Most common type (90% of all).
   Poor LV contraction.
   Familial in 25% patients.
   Other causes: Alcohol, beri-beri, Coxackie, Chagas disease, cocaine, doxorubicin, AZT.
   Features: Dyspnoea, oedema, fatigue, palpitations.
   Examination: Gallop rhythm (S3), tricuspid/ mitral regurgitation, progressive CHF, emboli, arrhythmia.
   Investigations: CXR, ECHO.
   Treatment: Treat CHF, A Fib (digoxin), ventricular tachycardia (Vtach) – cardioversion/ defibrillation.

2. *Hypertrophic cardiomyopathy.*
   Idiopathic (most common cause of sudden death in athletes).
   Troponin T and β myosin gene mutations.
   Reduced stroke volume (SV).
   Most cases familial, AD (autosomal dominant).
   Features: Sudden death, dyspnoea, angina, syncope, arrhythmias.
   Examination: LVH, systolic murmur, Vtach is a major cause of sudden death.
   Investigations: ECHO.
   Treatment: Beta blockers, calcium channel blockers, amiodarone.
   Internal defibrillator.
   Surgical resection.

3. *Restrictive cardiomyopathy*
   Diastolic filling restricted.
   Causes: Amyloidosis, sarcoidosis, hemochromatosis, scarring, fibrosis.
   Features: Dyspnoea, oedema, fatigue, palpitations.
   Examination: Progressive CHF, emboli, arrhythmia.
   Diagnosed by ECHO, catheterization, endomyocardial biopsy.
   Treatment: None, poor prognosis.

What does Irene's EF indicate?

The two-dimensional echocardiography demonstrated signs of chronic right ventricular pressure overload. Irene's anatomic compromise of the pulmonary vascular bed secondary to her lung disorder, COPD was the likely cause of her RHF. This increase in pulmonary arterial pressure because of increased pulmonary resistance, which is normally about 1/3 of TPR, is often seen in COPD. This can eventually lead to RVH and RHF. RVH secondary to lung disease is called *cor pulmonale.*

Back to John's exam . . .

Meanwhile let's return to Dr Smith's examination of John. His carotid pulses were equal with no bruits. His femoral pulses were reduced on the left, and his dorsalis pedis were impalpable on both feet and his posterior tibial pulses were reduced.

Which arteries are commonly palpated in a physical examination?
What is the significance of these clinical findings?
Which clinical conditions cause reduced foot pulses?

'I'm afraid you could be suffering from angina' Dr Smith told John. 'What this means is that your arteries are clogged up and can't deliver oxygen to the leg and heart muscles they supply. That is why you get leg pains and chest pains'.

'Why does it happen when I'm walking up Sunnybrook Hill?' John asked.

Dr Smith explained that the muscles need more oxygen when they are exercising and the blockage was preventing this.

'In order to climb Sunnybrook Hill your heart and calf muscles have to work harder,' Dr Smith said. 'So they need more oxygen. Unfortunately because of the blockages, your blood vessels cannot supply the extra oxygen to your muscles'.

'Can't you unblock them?' John asked.

What is the most likely cause of the blockages in John's arteries?

John's intermittent claudication allows us to review the circulatory system focussing initially on the coronary circulation, which is shown in Figure 2.13.

Which of the coronary arteries, if blocked, lead to the worst prognosis?

Let us now look at the circulatory system in general. You need to know the main arterial and venous vessels, which we will come across as we move through the different chapters. For now be able to correctly identify the following major blood vessels in a diagram (or in a cadaver if you have access to one!!). Get someone to test you and tick the boxes in Table 2.4!!

Draw cross-sectional diagrams of an artery, a vein and a capillary. Got to know your tunicas!!

John and Mary were watching a news item on TV. Air travel, the reporter was saying can cause clots in leg veins. Will the blocked blood vessels in my legs cause me problems when we fly off to Benidorm in the summer John wondered?

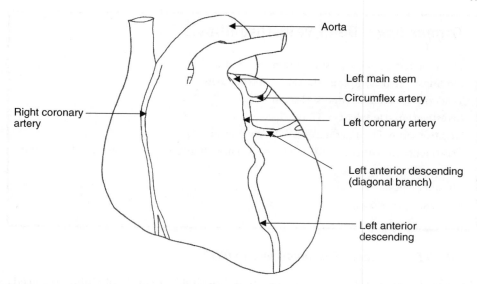

Figure 2.13 Coronary arterial circulation. Adapted from Kumar and Clark(2006) Clinical Medicine 5th ED Saunders.

Table 2.4 Major blood vessels

Vessel	Correctly identified
Internal and external *carotid* arteries	
Jugular vein	
Subclavian artery and vein	
Axillary artery	
Brachial artery	
Radial artery	
Ulnar artery	
Antecubital vein	
Basilar and cephalic veins	
Azygous vein	
Intercostal veins	
Ascending and descending aorta	
Coeliac trunk and its branches	
Splenic artery and vein	
Hepatic, hepatic portal vein and hepatic veins	
Renal artery and veins	
Inferior and superior vena cava (IVC and SVC)	
Superior and inferior mesenteric artery (SMA, IMA)	
Pudendal arteries	
Femoral artery	
Poplitial artery	
Saphenous vein	
Dorsalis pedias artery	
Posterial tibial artery	

Trigger box   **Deep vein thrombosis**

Thrombi in deep veins most commonly in the leg.
Findings: Often asymptomatic, calf pain tenderness.
Tenderness, swelling, redness, Homan's sign.
Investigation: Doppler US.
Negative serum D-Dimer makes DVT very unlikely.
Treatment: All patients with DVT above knee should be anticoagulated to prevent pulmonary embolism.
Thrombolytics.
Elastic support stockings.

?   *Which factors/conditions predispose to DVT?*

'I'm afraid I have to refer you to Dr Hart at the hospital,' Dr Smith told John. 'We need to confirm my diagnosis and then find out the extent of the blockages. In the meantime I'll prescribe some GTN spray for the chest pain.'

?   *How does GTN relieve anginal pain? What is its MOA?*

John posed a question. 'What about my BP Doc?'
   John had been suffering from hypertension for several years. It was picked up on one of his rare visits to the surgery.
   'Well, it's a little high today,' Dr Smith replied – his BP was 150/97.
   'What's causing this high blood pressure?' John asked Dr Smith.
   'In most of cases we don't know,' Dr Smith replied.

   Let us have a look at the important concept of blood pressure.
   Blood pressure (mean arterial pressure) is worked out from the formula shown below:

$$MAP = DP + PP/3$$

Where PP = SP-DP
   BP is a product of two variables and is shown in the formula shown below:
   BP = CO × TPR
   MAP, mean arterial pressure; DP, diastolic pressure; PP, pulse pressure; SP, systolic pressure; CO, cardiac output; TPR, total peripheral resistance.

R (single vessel) ∞ $1/r^4$
Where R is resistance and r is radius of vessel.

One day Irene fainted while standing up from a sitting position. Dr Smith explained that this can happen to elderly people.
   'When you stand up suddenly,' he said 'the blood pools in the veins in your legs due to gravity. Your BP falls and you don't get enough blood and therefore oxygen going to your brain, so you faint.'

'This is called orthostatic hypotension. In elderly people there is reduced baroreceptor responsiveness, and the decreased arterial compliance causes the problem.'

How do you diagnose orthostatic hypertension? What other conditions can cause orthostatic hypotension?

Regulation of BP is shown in Figure 2.14.

Short-term regulation (Fig. 2.14a) uses the autonomic nervous system and responses occur within seconds. The *vasomotor centre* activates the sympathetic nervous system to increase BP by: (i) increasing heart rate and cardiac contractility; (ii) inducing arteriolar vasoconstriction (except in muscles), which increases peripheral vascular resistance; (iii) increasing venous return by inducing a venoconstriction; (iv) stimulating the release of sympathetic catecholamines from the adrenal medulla.

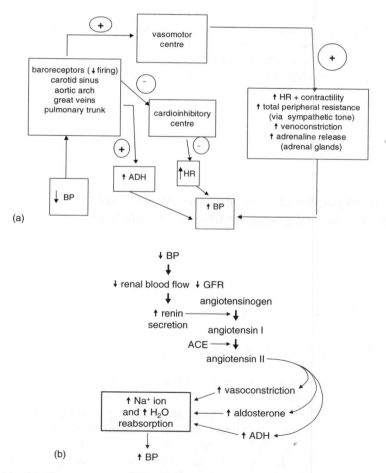

Figure 2.14 (a) Short-term regulation of blood pressure (ADH = antidiuretic hormone). (b) Long-term regulation of blood pressure (ACE = angiotensin converting enzyme)

The *cardioinhibitory centre* activates the parasympathetic nervous system to reduce heart rate. Little effect is seen on venous return or peripheral resistance.

Note the reflexes modulating the autonomic nervous system. An increase in BP causes an increased stretch of baroreceptors in the carotid sinus and aortic arch, which inhibits the vasomotor centre and stimulates the cardioinhibitory centre to reduce BP. The increasing blood volume also increases cardiopulmonary barore-ceptor stretch in the great veins, atria and pulmonary trunk. This decreases vaso-constrictor sympathetic activity and the release of antidiuretic hormone (ADH), so decreases cardiac output and total peripheral resistance. Opposite responses are seen when there is a decrease in BP.

If BP falls, low oxygenation activates peripheral chemoreceptors in aortic and carotid bodies, which stimulate vasoconstrictor sympathetic nerves, so increasing BP.

In *cerebral ischaemia*, low BP results in the accumulation of CO_2 and H^+ ions in the brain, so stimulating the vasomotor centre to increase BP.

The *Cushing reflex* is seen when a rise in intracranial pressure compresses cerebral arteries and so reduces blood flow. Stimulation of sympathetic nerves raises arterial BP above intracranial pressure to restore blood flow.

The renin–angiotensin system requires several hours for effects to occur (Fig. 2.14b). Here changes in renal blood flow cause changes in Na^+ ion and water excretion.

What is the function of atrial natriuretic protein (ANP)?
What is the Valsalva procedure? What is its significance?

  List the main causes of syncope.

John suffers from essential hypertension. Table 2.5 shows the types of hypertension, their causes and consequences.

Since $BP = CO \times TPR$, raised BP can be controlled by reducing CO or TPR. Table 2.6 shows the common treatment strategies used in the treatment of hypertension.

'Make an appointment with the practice nurse for some fasting blood tests and come and see me a week later. The results should be in by then,' Dr Smith said as John rose to leave.

Table 2.5 Types of hypertension, their causes and consequences

Essential hypertension (95% of hypertensive patients)	
	Unknown cause. Probably multifactorial aetiology. Genetic, fetal, humoral, insulin resistance and environmental factors. Obesity, alcohol intake, sodium intake and stress are significant contributing factors.
Secondary hypertension (5% of hypertensive patients)	
Renal causes	80% of secondary hypertension. Common causes are diabetic nephropathy, chronic glomerulonephritis, adult polycystic kidney disease, chronic tubulointerstitial nephritis, and renovascular disease.
Endocrine causes	Conn's syndrome, adrenal hyperplasia, phaeochromocytoma, Cushing's syndrome, acromegaly.
Cardiovascular causes	Coarctation of aorta.
Drugs	Oral contraceptive pill (OCP), steroids, carbenoxolone, vasopressin, monoamine oxidase inhibitor(MAOI) + tyramine-containing foods.
Pregnancy	Pre-eclampsia and eclampsia
Consequences	Increased risk of cardiovascular events.
	Haemorrhagic stroke and atherothrombotic strokes.
	Cardiac death due to coronary events or cardiac failure.
	Peripheral arterial disease. Associated risk increased by 2×
Malignant hypertension	BP rises rapidly. Diastolic BP > 140 mmHg, 1-year survival <20% if not treated.

Table 2.6 Drug treatment in hypertension

Drug class	Drug examples	Mechanism of action	Side-effects
Thiazide diuretics	Bendroflumethiazide	Inhibit distal tubule Na/Cl symporters, so reducing reabsorption	Hypokalaemia, hyponatraemia, hypomagnesaemia, hypercalcaemia, hyperuricaemia, hyperglycaemia, altered plasma lipid levels, alkalosis.

(Continued)

Table 2.6 (*Continued*)

Drug class	Drug examples	Mechanism of action	Side-effects
Beta blockers	Propranolol, atenolol	Initially reduces heart rate and cardiac output, but with chronic use cardiac output returns, as peripheral resistance may have been reset at a lower level to keep BP low. Reduced renin release.	Bronchospasm, bradycardia, impotence, fatigue
Centrally acting α_2-adrenergic agonists	Methyldopa, clonidine	Reduce sympathetic tone by stimulating central alpha$_2$-adrenoceptors	Bradycardia, postural hypotension, headache, dizziness, nocturnal unrest/ nightmares, impotence, mild psychosis, impaired mental acuity, hepatitis, jaundice, pancreatitis, haemolytic anaemia
α_1-adrenergic blockers	Doxasozin, Prazosin, terazosin	Causes vasodilatation by blocking α_1-receptors in peripheral blood vessels.	Orthostasis
Ca^{2+} channel blockers	Nifedipine, felodipine, dilitiazem, verapamil	Blocks L-type Ca^{2+} ion channels, so decreases vascular smooth muscle tone causing vasodilatation	Vasodilators
Hydralazine, minoxidil	Dilates arterioles and arteries, so decreasing afterload	Hydralazine – lupus like syndrome, compensatory tachycardia.	Dizziness, flushing, ankle oedema, hypotension Minoxidil – orthostasis, facial hirsutism
ACE inhibitors	Ramipril, captopril, enalapril	Inhibits the conversion of angiotensin I to angiotensin II. Angiotensin is a potent vasoconstrictor and also stimulates the release of aldosterone	Hypotension (especial on first dose), dry cough (due to brady- kinin accumulation), hyperkalaemia, angioedema, rash
Angiotensin II receptor antagonists	Losartan, valsartan	Antagonizes the angiotensin II receptor	Rashes, leukopenia, hyperkalaemia

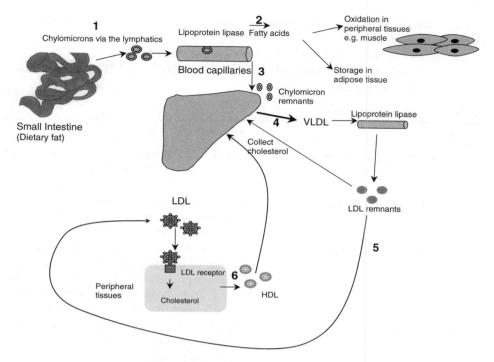

Figure 2.15 Lipoprotein transport

John spent the next week in a state of anxiety. He was worried about the impending hospital visit and what the blood tests might reveal.

He was fifteen minutes early for his appointment at the surgery. Dr Smith had more bad news.

'I'm afraid your cholesterol levels are high.' he announced dryly.

The different lipoproteins involved are shown in Table 2.7. Lipoprotein transport is shown in Figure 2.15. Can you describe stages 1–6?

Table 2.7 Lipoproteins

Low density lipoprotein (LDL): is formed from VLDL in the circulation and transports cholesterol to the peripheral tissues and is also taken up by the liver.

High density lipoprotein (HDL): transports cholesterol from the peripheral tissues to the liver where it is metabolized.

Chylomicrons (CM): transports exogenous (dietary) lipids (mainly triglycerides and some cholesterol) from the gut to the peripheral tissues (mainly triglycerides) and liver (mainly cholesterol).

Very low density lipoproteins (VLDL): transport endogenous lipid (mainly triglycerides but also some cholesterol) from the liver to the peripheral tissues.

High cholesterol levels can be found in dyslipidaemias. Table 2.8 shows the key types of dyslipidaemia.

Dr Smith prescribed some statins for John's raised cholesterol.

'Your hospital appointment should come in a few weeks,' he said. 'Then we will have a full picture of your angina'.

Table 2.8   The dyslipidaemias

Disease	Features
Familial dysbetalipoproteinaemia	Raised LDL and triglyceride levels due to raised IDLs and chylomicron remnants. Associated with obesity and glucose intolerance.
Familial combined hyperlipidaemia	Raised cholesterol and triglyceride levels, which carries an increased risk of coronary artery disease.
Familial hypercholesterolaemia	Raised LDL levels and mild elevation of triglycerides. Heterozygotes often develop coronary artery disease. Homozygotes have very high cholesterol levels and have an early onset of coronary artery disease.
Familial hypertriglyceridaemia	Raised VLDL levels associated with diabetes and exacerbated by excessive alcohol consumption, obesity and glucocorticoids.
Lipoprotein lipase deficiency	Rare condition characterized by a lack of chylomicron metabolism. Childhood hepatospenomegaly commonly results.

Treatment of hyperlipidaemia is shown in Table 2.9.

 Find out the mechanisms of acion of bile acids and niacin.

Table 2.9   Treatment of hyperlipidaemia

Drug	Therapeutic effects	Toxicity
HMG-COA reductase inhibitors (simvastatin, pravastatin)	Decreases LDL-C +++ Increases HDL-C + Decreases TG +	LFT s increase, myositis
Bile acid resins (cholestyramine, colestipol)	Decreases LDL-C ++ Increases TG +	GI discomfort
Niacin	Decreases LDL-C ++ Increases HDL-C ++ Decreases TG +	Flushing
Lipoprotein lipase inhibitors(gemfibrozil)	Decreases LDL-C + Increases HDL-C+ Decreases TG +++	LFT s increase, myositis

+ Degree of effect.

Figure 2.16 shows how the atheroma in John's arteries developed.

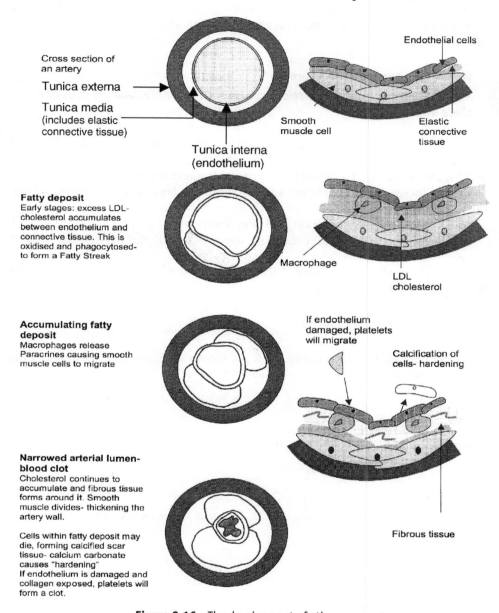

Figure 2.16 The development of atheroma

Dr Smith had more bad news for John.
'Your blood sugar level is a bit higher than normal,' he said.
'So am I diabetic as well?' John asked sullenly.

Dr Smith shook his head. 'Not yet. You might have what we call impaired glucose tolerance. We have to do a test called an oral glucose tolerance test, an OGTT, to diagnose this condition. So while you are not diabetic as such, you could be heading that way.'

What is impaired glucose tolerance?
Atherosclerosis can lead to aortic aneurysms. Describe the common sites where these occur.

John's appointment at the cardiology centre arrived 3 weeks later. Dr Hart had ordered an exercise ECG test. John felt confident; he had heard that it just involved walking on a treadmill. He was in for a surprise! It was easy to begin with but then the technician increased the incline and speeded things up. Soon John was running. Then the chest pains came.

John's exercise test had to be stopped after 5 minutes.

John wanted to carry on. The chest pains weren't that bad. But the technician didn't agree.

'Your ECG is showing horizontal ST depression in several leads.' she said curtly helping him off the treadmill.

Describe the Bruce protocol.

The ECG findings in John's exercise test are shown in Figure 2.17. Features of the different types of angina are shown in Table 2.10.

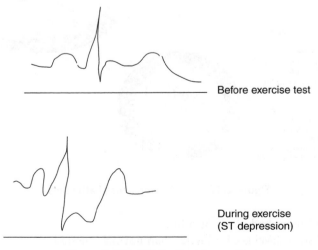

Before exercise test

During exercise
(ST depression)

Figure 2.17   ECG findings in angina

Table 2.10 Angina types

Classic angina pectoris	Angina on exertion. Standard medical anti-anginal therapy (beta blockers and nitrates).
Decubitus angina	Occurs on lying down. Impaired LV function.
Nocturnal angina	Provoked by vivid dreams.
Variant (Prinzmetal's) angina	Angina at rest without provocation. Due to vasospasm.
Cardiac syndrome X	Positive exercise tolerance test but normal coronary angiography. Difficult to treat.
Unstable angina (acute coronary syndrome)	Worsening angina or angina at rest. A medical emergency, requiring hospital admission for bed rest, oxygen, morphine, aspirin, clopidogrel and standard medical anti-anginal therapy. Angiography and coronary revascularization. Percutaneous transluminal coronary angioplasty (PTCA), coronary artery bypass grafting (CABG).

What is the pathophysiology of unstable angina?

Later that morning John met Dr Hart. Dr Hart informed him that he would have to return to the hospital for more tests.

'We have to do a coronary angiogram to assess which arteries are blocked,' he said. 'Hopefully we should be able to get you a slot in a few weeks'

'What happens if they are blocked, Doc?' John asked.

'Well that depends on the extent of the blockages and the general state of your coronary circulation,' Dr Hart replied. 'You may have to be treated medically, you may need angioplasty or a bypass graft.'

> An equivocal exercise test may require carrying out a technitium perfusion scan. Describe the principles underlying myocardial perfusion scanning. Why is (a) adenosine, (b) dobutamine used?

John's little elephant...

John was sitting at home watching TV. It was two weeks since his visit to Dr Hart and he hadn't heard from the hospital about the date for his angiogram. It had been a particularly stressful day at work with an unpleasant meeting where redundancies were mentioned. He had come home tense. After wolfing down his food and washing it down with two cans of beer he settled down on the sofa.

Around 8 pm he began to sweat and he felt nauseous. Then came the pain. It was like his angina but a hundred times worse. It was a like a little elephant sitting on his chest he would describe later. The pain went down his left arm and his left jaw began to hurt as well. Mary rang for an ambulance.

The paramedics were at the house in five minutes. They found a pale looking John clutching his chest; sweating profusely. One of the paramedics quickly hooked him up to an oxygen cylinder while the other fired off some questions. 'How bad is the pain? Does it change with breathing or movement? Does it run down your left arm or up to the jaw? How long have you had the pain? Can you describe it? Any history of heart trouble?'

? ***What is the significance of all these questions?***

The paramedics gave him GTN, placed him in a trolley and took him into the ambulance. Soon, the ambulance, its blue light flashing and siren wailing, was speeding towards Hope hospital. Inside one of the paramedics hooked John up to a portable ECG machine. His ECG showed ST elevations in leads V3 andV4 consistent with occlusion of the LAD artery. Johns BP was190/110 pulse 80. They gave him morphine and an aspirin.

? ***What is the basis of these treatments?***

John arrived at the hospital some 10 minutes later. The chest pains were much less; the morphine was certainly working.

The Emergency Doctors were waiting for him. John was examined and subsequent ECGs confirmed an anterior myocardial infarction (Figure 2.18). Types of MI are shown in Table 2.11.

Suddenly John lost consciousness.' He's in Vtach' one of the nurses shouted. A doctor placed a defibrillator on John's chest and administered an electric shock. Luckily the tachycardia returned to a normal sinus rhythm and John regained consciousness a few minutes later.

? ***Why was John defibrillated?***

Table 2.11 Types of MI

Location	Coronary artery affected	Changes in leads
Septal MI	Left coronary: left anterior descending (LAD)–Septal branch	V1 to V3
Anterior MI	Left coronary: LAD–diagonal branch	V2- V5
Inferior MI	Right coronary: posterior descending branch	II, III, aVF
Lateral MI	Left coronary: circumflex branch	V5, V6, I, AVL
RV MI	Right coronary: proximal branch	V4R (lead V4 placed on right chest)

Note: Non ST elevation myocardial infarctions (NSTEMI) refer to myocardial infarction without ST segment elevation. Grouped with unstable angina under acute coronary syndrome.

Trigger box   Common arrhythmias

1. *Paroxysmal supraventricular tachycardia (PSVT)*
Mechanisms: Re-entry circuit between atria and ventricles, between atrium and AV node.
Features: palpitations, angina, SOB, heart rate (HR): 150–250,
ECG: Normal QRS, P wave may be buried.
Treatment: vagotonic manoeuvres (e.g. carotid massage, Valsalva), adenosine, radiofrequency ablation.

2. *Atrial fibrillation*
Mechanism: spontaneous rapid atrial depolarization (300/min). Refractory AV node limits conduction to ventricles.
Causes: CHD, thyrotoxicosis, RF, COPD, alcohol, sepsis.
Features: Irregularly irregular pulse, often asymptomatic, SOB, palpitations, chest pain.
ECG: No P wave, irregular and variable QRS.
Treatment: Anticoagulation, Calcium channel blockers, digoxin, beta blockers, cardio-version.

3. *Atrial flutter*
Mechanism: Circular circuit around atrium (300/min). Conduction to ventricles limited to every second, third or fourth depolarization.
Causes: CHD, COPD, pericarditis, valvular disease.
Features: Pulse 150(2:1), 100(3:1), 75(4:1) regular, asymptomatic, palpitations, syncope.
ECG: Regular sawtooth P waves,
Treatment: Drugs as in AF, anticoagulation, radiofrequency ablation.

4. *Premature ventricular tachycardia (PVT)*
Mechanisms: Ventricular foci giving rise to ectopic beats.
Causes: Hypoxia, hyperthyroidism, electrolyte abnormalities.
Features: Often asymptomatic, palpitations.
ECG: Early wide QRS (no preceding P wave), compensatory pause.
Treatment: None, beta blocker if symptomatic

5. *Ventricular tachycardia (VT)*
Mechanism: Rapid ventricular depolarizations due to re-entrant circuits, ventricular myocardium showing abnormal triggered activity.
Causes: MI, drugs, electrolyte abnormalities, long QT syndrome.
Features: Non-sustained VT – often asymptomatic, sustained VT – palpitations, angina, hypotension, progression to VF.
ECG: 3+ PVCs, Wide QRS regular rhythm, AV dissociation.
Treatment: Amiodarone, lidocaine, cardioversion, ICDs.

6. *Ventricular fibrillation (VF)*

Mechanism: ventricular ectopic activity.

Causes: MI.

Features: With or without pulse, syncope, hypotension.
ECG erratic pattern.

Treatment: Immediate cardioversion.

Some bloods were drawn and sent to monitor for cardiac enzymes and John was treated with streptokinase and a beta-blocker. Details of the cardiac enzymes used in the investigation of acute MI are shown in Table 2.12 and Figure 2.19.

John was thrombolysed. Note the post thrombolytic ECG trace in Figure 2.18. Thrombolytic therapy and the pathway involved are shown in Table 2.13 and Figure 2.20. Figure 2.21 shows the histopathological changes in John's heart following his MI.

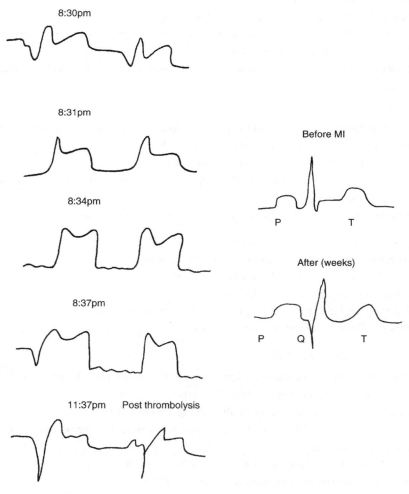

Figure 2.18   Changes in lead III during John's acute MI

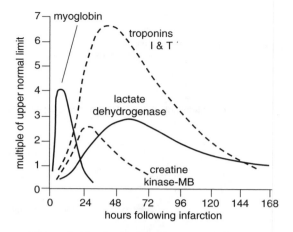

Figure 2.19 Cardiac enzymes post infarction

Table 2.12 Cardiac enzymes

Serum Troponins (I or T): highly sensitive and specific markers of myocardial damage.

Myoglobin: sensitive marker of myocardial damage but non-specific and released following skeletal muscle damage.

Serum CK-MB: levels rise within 3–6 hours of myocardial damage; peak by about 12–24 hours and return to baseline within 24–48 hours.

Serum aspartate aminotransferase (AST) and lactate dehyrogenase (LDH): rarely of value in the diagnosis and management of myocardial infarction.

N.B. These tests are often done in combination and serially. Serum myoglobin and CK-MB, if normal within 6-10 hours of the onset of chest pain are useful in excluding myocardial infarction. Serum troponins are useful in confirming myocardial damage and diagnosing myocardial infarction in patients presenting after 24 hours.

Table 2.13 Thrombolytic therapy

Thrombolytics
Streptokinase
Tissue-type plasminogen activator (t-PA).

Thrombolytic therapy improves survival rates in myocardial infarction (MI).

'Door-to-drug' time should be <30 minutes. Given within the first 2 hours may abort MI

Administer thrombolytics ASAP up to 12 hours from symptom onset in patients with ST-segment elevation >1 mm in two or more anatomically contiguous ECG leads, new or presumed new left bundle-branch block, or anterior ST depression where posterior infarction is suspected, or high serum cardiac markers.

Absolute contraindications: Stroke or active bleeding in last 2 months, systolic BP > 200 mmHg, proliferative diabetic retinopathy, pregnancy.

Relative contraindications: prolonged or traumatic resuscitation, recent surgery or trauma, known bleeding tendencies or current use of anticoagulants.

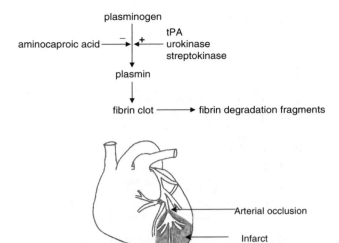

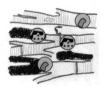

Figure 2.20   Drugs affecting the fibrinolytic system

1) 8-24 hours

Small infiltration of neutrophils
Separation of fibres

2) 1-3 days- pallor

Extensive coagulative necrosis
Fibres have lost striations
Infiltration of neutrophils and macrophages

3) 3-10 days- yellowing and
softening

Ingrowth of granulation tissue with leukocytes
still present

4) Weeks- months

Scar tissue complete (may have living muscle
fibres embedded)

Figure 2.21   The evolution of myocardial infarction

The next day John was transferred to the coronary care ward. Angiography later confirmed blockage in the LAD and RCA and John was offered coronary artery bypass graft surgery (CABG).

Compare and contrast angioplasty and CABG.

? *What is Dressler's syndrome?*

3

The gastrointestinal system

Learning strategy

The gastrointestinal tract (GIT) is basically a tube where different regions carry out various functions involving the process of digestion and absorption.

A good way to learn the key facts and concepts of the GIT is to start from the mouth and work your way downward. The storyline attempts to do this by considering clinical scenarios involving some common conditions affecting different parts of the GIT. As you read these scenarios, you can revise the normal anatomy, embryology, physiology and biochemistry relevant to the regions and the structures found within them. In addition to considering the pathophysiology of the GIT we will also cover the mechanisms of action of the key drugs used in GI medicine.

Try to answer the questions and try to complete the Learning tasks.

Mary's burning stomach...

For as long as she can remember, Mary had 'tummy problems'. She had suffered from regular attacks of heartburn, bloating and diarrhoea, which came on especially when she had a bad attack of 'nerves'. She had managed her discomforts with antacids. John's illnesses had made things worse and her complaints became much more frequent.

Her first serious problem began in July, some 6 months after John's heart attack. She went to see Dr Smith with a 'burning' sensation in the middle of her abdomen for the past 2 days. She described the pain as moderately severe but did not mention any radiation. She had also vomited.

History revealed that the pain seemed to be relieved a little by eating and by taking her regular antacid. Mary also mentioned that she had been feeling lethargic and weak for

Integrated Medical Sciences by Shantha Perera, Stephen Anderson, Ho Leung and Rousseau Gama
© 2007 John Wiley & Sons, Ltd ISBN: 978470016589 (HB) 978470016596 (PB)

weeks. Her bowel functions were abnormal and she had passed black tarry stools three days previously.

Dr Smith examined her. He found her abdomen soft and non-distended but detected some mild epigastric tenderness. No hepatosplenomegaly or masses were found. Rectal examination found no masses and no obvious blood. He weighed her and checked her records: there was no history of weight loss.

Dr Smith arranged a blood test. The results arrived a week later. Mary's full blood count showed a low Hb of 9.1 g/dl (NR 12.0–16.0) with the rest of the parameters being within normal limits.

What do you think is the most likely cause of her low haemoglobin?

Clearly Mary's problem involved the gastrointestinal (GI) system, which we are going to consider in this chapter.

Let us begin by considering the key developmental issues. First, in terms of origins, the GI tract is endodermal and begins as a primitive gut tube. The primitive gut tube is divided into the foregut, the midgut and the hindgut. The derivatives of these regions are shown in Figure 3.1.

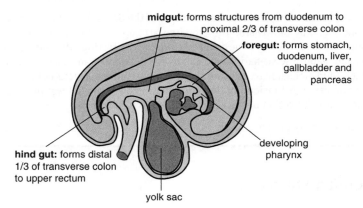

Figure 3.1   The derivatives of the fore, mid and hindgut (around 28 days). Adapted from Tortora and Grabowski (2003), Principles of Anatomy and Physiology, 10th edition, John Wiley & Sons

As mentioned in Chapter 1 an outgrowth of the foregut gives rise to the respiratory system. In the 4th week the oesophagotracheal septum separates the foregut into the respiratory diverticulum (lung bud) and oesophagus. A tracheosophagal fistula can however be present if this process does not take place properly (Figure 3.2).

Physiological herniation starts at week 6 and the gut returns at week 10. Important abnormalities that can occur include malrotation of the midgut, stenosis and duplications. There can also be remnants of the vitelline duct, which can lead to the problem seen in Figure 3.3.

What are the features of Meckel's diverticulum?

Other problems include an annular pancreas and rectal atresia.

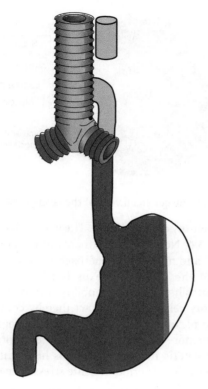

Figure 3.2 Tracheoesophageal fistula

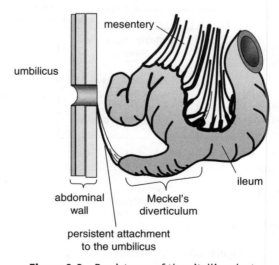

Figure 3.3 Persistence of the vitelline duct

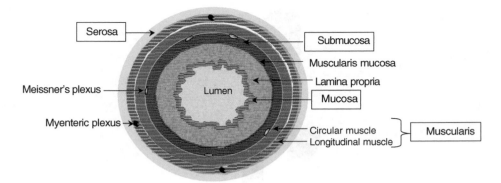

Figure 3.4   The general layout of the layers forming the GIT

Let us now review the anatomy of the GI tract. The general layout of the layers of the GI tract is shown in Figure 3.4. Note the components of the enteric nervous system; the submucosal (Meissner's) and myenteric (Auerbach's) plexuses.

The main function of the myentric plexus is to supply motor neurons to the musculature thereby controlling GI tract mobility. Motor neurons of the Meissner's plexus supply the secretory cells of the GI tract thereby controlling secretions. Interneurons connect the two plexuses. Additionally, sensory neurons supply the mucosal epithelium acting as chemoreceptors and stretch receptors.The close relationship between the central and enteric nervous systems is highlighted by Mary's diarrhoea, which seems to come on during a period of acute stress. The enteric nervous system is shown in Figure 3.5.

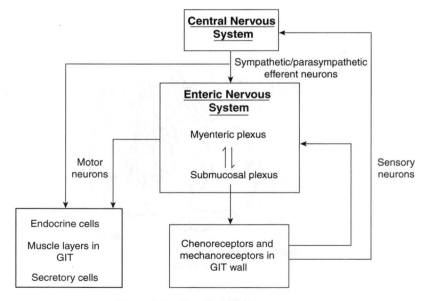

Figure 3.5   The enteric nervous system

Review the anatomy of the important structures found in the head, the salivary glands, teeth, oropharynx, epiglottis.

 Outline the key physiological functions of saliva.

 What are the causes of parotitis?

When Dr Smith examined Mary, he palpated the abdomen. Figure 3.6 shows the abdominal regions and indicates underlying organs. You should know the general gross features of the organs, their relationships to other structures, their blood and nerve supply and their key histological features.

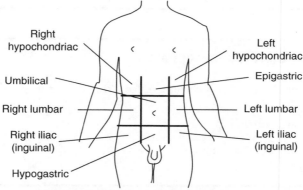

- **Right hypochondriac:** right liver lobe.
- **Right lumbar:** gallbladder and ascending colon.
- **Right iliac:** caecum and appendix.
- **Epigastric:** left liver lobe and stomach.
- **Umbilical:** small intestines and transverse colon.
- **Hypogastric:** urinary bladder.
- **Left hypochondriac:** stomach.
- **Left lumbar:** descending colon.
- **Left iliac:** initial portion of the sigmoid colon.

Figure 3.6 Abdominal regions and the underlying organs

Mary periodically suffers from heartburn. This could be due to gastroesophageal reflux disease (GORD) where stomach acid refluxes back into the oesophagus.

This allows us to look at the oesophagus. Things you need to know include, the upper oesophageal sphincter (UOS) the lower oesophageal sphincter (LOS), the types of tissue making up the inner lining, and the types of muscle found along the length of the oesophagus.

 Describe the mechanism of swallowing.

GORD is most commonly due to an incompetent relaxation of the LOS. Another cause can be a hiatal hernia.

What are the risk factors associated with GORD?

Trigger box   Achalasia

Unknown aetiology.
Risk factor for oesophageal cancer.
Pathology: Decrease of ganglionic cells in oesophageal wall, vagal degeneration. LOS fails
to relax, aperistalsis.
Features: Dysphagia (solids and liquids), regurgitation, chest pain, chest infections.
Investigations: Barium swallow (beak deformity), oesophageal manometry.
Treatment: Endoscopic pneumatic dilatation of LOS.

Trigger box   Barrett's oesophagus

Pathology: Stratified squamous epithelium replaced with columnar epithelium.
Due to reflux.
Predisposes to adenocarcinoma.

What are the features of this condition?
How is it treated?

Trigger box   Hiatal hernia

Diagnosed by barium swallow or oesophagogastroduodenoscopy (OGD).

1. *Sliding type* (95%)
    Gastro-oesophageal junction slides through hiatus.
    Presents as GORD.
    Treatment: Medical – as for GORD.

2. *Para-oesophageal* (5%)
    Section of stomach moves through hiatus.
    Gastro-oesophageal junction below diaphragm.
    Treatment: Surgical gastropexy.

Mary's stomach problems eventually took her to hospital. Further investigations
revealed that Mary was suffering from peptic ulcer disease caused by *Helicobacter pylori*.
This will allow us to move a bit further down the GI tract into the stomach.

Trigger box H. pylori

Gram-negative, urease producer.

Found in gastric antrum, duodenum.

Associated with chronic active gastritis, peptic ulcer disease (PUD), gastric cancer, gastric lymphoma.

Investigations: Urease test, Gram stain and culture, urea breath test, serology, stool detection test.

Trigger box Peptic ulcer disease

Stomach, duodenum, and lower oesophagus; after gastric surgery it involves the gastro-enterostomy stoma.

Duodenum most common site.

Mucosal damage caused by compromised mucosal defence and/or increased acid and pepsin. High H^+ concentration can disrupt protective mechanisms of the mucosal barrier.

Duodenal ulcer: Usually high basal acid output and normal serum gastrin.

Gastric ulcer: Normal or slightly low acid secretion.

Nearly all duodenal ulcers and most gastric ulcers not associated with non-steroidal anti-inflammatory drugs (NSAIDs) are caused by *H. pylori*.

Helicobacter infection of the mucosa impairs the protective mechanisms and allows secondary damage from the acid environment.

Epigastric pain is caused by the inflammatory reaction to chemical (HCl and pepsin) injury to the mucosa.

Bleeding is caused by erosion of the submucosa exposing underlying blood vessels.

Damage to the deeper muscle layers of the wall can lead to fibrosis and ischaemia.

Erosion through the serosal surface causes sudden severe epigastric pain and life-threatening peritonitis.

Chronic ulcers in the pyloric region and duodenum can cause obstruction to the outlet of the stomach because of the narrow lumen, leading to profuse vomiting.

Treatment: Omeprazole, metronidazole, clarithromycin.

Figure 3.7 shows the main anatomical features of the stomach. Note the extra muscle layer, the body, fundus and the pylorus. Understand the significance of pyloric sphincter. The vagus supplies the parasympathetic nerve supply to the stomach.

Before the introduction of H_2 receptor antagonists and proton-pump inhibitors, vagotomy helped in the management of severe peptic ulcer disease.

What was the rationale of this treatment strategy?

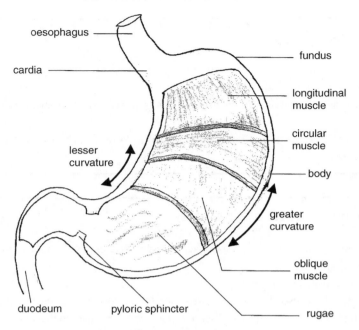

Figure 3.7   Stomach anatomy

Mary's melaena suggests that a blood vessel may have eroded due to the ulcer. This gives us a chance to consider the blood supply to the stomach as seen in Figure 3.8. The gastroduodenal artery is commonly damaged in PUD.

Trigger box   **Gastritis**

Inflammation of the stomach.

Features: Often asymptomatic, indigestion, haematemesis, melaena, nausea, vomiting.

Endoscopy for diagnosis.

Treatment: depends on aetiology.

1. *Acute gastritis*
   Causes: NSAIDs, alcohol, burns, CNS disease.

2. *Chronic gastritis*
   Type A (10%)
   Can lead to pernicious anaemia (what is the mechanism?)
   Found in the fundus.
   Type B (90%)
   Caused by NSAIDs, *H. pylori.*
   Increased risk of PUD, gastric cancer.

How is gastritis managed?

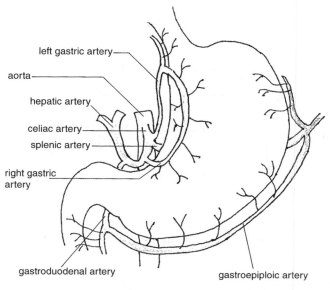

left gastric artery

aorta

hepatic artery

celiac artery

splenic artery

right gastric artery

gastroduodenal artery

gastroepiploic artery

Figure 3.8   Blood supply to the stomach

Trigger box   **Gastric cancer**

Adenocarcinoma.

Features: Asymptomatic initially, abdominal pain, satiety, weight loss, epigastric mass, Virchow's node (where is it found?). Poor prognosis.

Investigations: Barium meal, gastroscopy, biopsy.

CT/MRI for staging.

Types

1. *Intestinal type*
   Risk factors: Nitrites, salt, low antioxidants, *H. pylori*, chronic gastritis.

2. *Diffuse type*
   More in men.
   Unknown risk factors.
   Treatment: surgery.

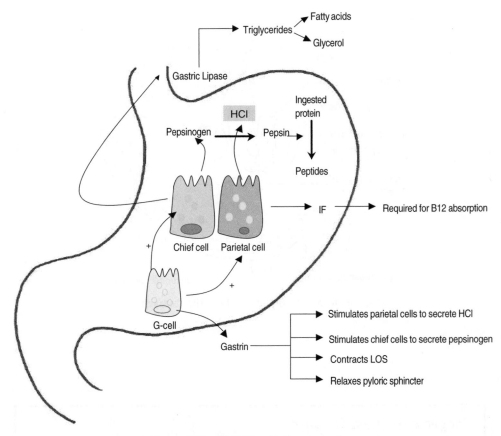

Figure 3.9   Digestion in the stomach

The digestive functions of the stomach can also be considered here. Figure 3.9 shows the digestion that takes place in the stomach. Note the different products secreted by the chief and parietal cells. Figure 3.10 shows the key triggers causing secretion of gastric juice. Note the role of acetylcholine (Ach), gastrin and histamine in causing secretion of H^+ ions.

Mary was prescribed a proton pump inhibitor (PPI) that decreases acid secretion. Note that gastrinomas can also produce excess acid. Table 3.1 shows the important drugs that are used to block peptic acid secretion.

List the main side effects of these drugs.

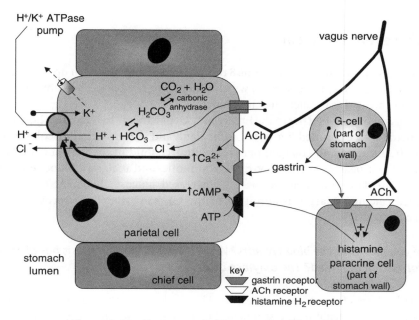

Figure 3.10 Factors controlling gastric acid secretion

Trigger box **Zollinger–Ellison syndrome**

Gastrinomas from G cells of pancreas.

Secretes gastrin.

25–50% associated with multiple endocrine neoplasia (MEN) type 1.

Features: Pain, diarrhoea, GI bleeding, weight loss, peptic ulcers.

Treatment: High dose PPI.

Surgery curative.

Can be resistant to treatment.

Table 3.1 Drugs used to block gastric acid secretion

Drug class	Mechanism of action
1. H_2-receptor antagonists: cimetidine, famotidine, nizatidine, ranitidine	Reducing gastric acid output as a result of histamine H_2-receptor blockade
2. PPIs: esomeprazole, lansoprazole, omeprazole, pantoprazole, rabeprazole	Inhibit gastric acid by blocking the H^+/K^+-ATPase enzyme system (the 'proton pump') of the gastric parietal cell
3. Prostaglandin analogues: misoprostol,	Antisecretory and protective properties.

Mary's severe backache ...

Mary's second problem occurred some 8 months later. She was woken up one night with abrupt onset severe epigastric pain, which radiated to her back. She vomited and was feeling very weak. John called the ambulance.

The paramedics rushed her to the Emergency Department (ED) at Hope hospital. The duty doctor who examined her noted some flank and periumbilical discoloration. An ultrasound indicated an enlarged pancreas with free fluid in the peritoneum. She was treated with nasogastric suction, i.v. fluids, antibiotics and analgesia. Blood tests showed increased amylase and lipase as well as increased glucose, LDH, AST, WBC, and decreased calcium. Mary was admitted to the GI ward where she recovered after 1 week and was discharged.

Can you interpret the blood results? What is your initial diagnosis based on the information provided? The amylase could be a clue ...

Mary had suffered from acute pancreatitis. This leads us to consider the functions of the GI structures just distal to the stomach. Figure 3.11 shows the major features of the pancreas and the duodenum and also shows the relationships of these organs to the liver and gall bladder.

Describe the pathophysiological mechanisms responsible for Mary's pancreatitis symptoms.

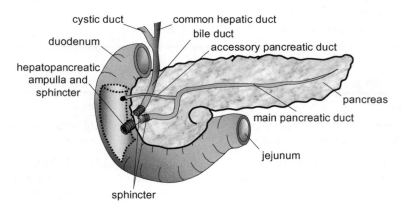

Figure 3.11   Anatomy of the pancreas and the duodenum

Trigger box   **Pancreatitis**

1. *Acute pancreatitis*

   Acinar cell injury: inflammation caused by gallstones, alcohol, drugs (steroids, azathioprine), metabolic (hypertriglyceridaemia, hypercalcaemia), infection (mumps), idiopathic.

   Features: Abdominal pain radiating to back or shoulder, tenderness, guarding, Cullen's sign, Grey Turner's sign.

   Increased amylase and lipase.

   Sentinel loop, colon cut-off sign on abdominal X-ray (AXR).

   Treatment: Analgesia, nasogastric (Ng) suction.

   Complications: Hyperglycemia, hypocalcemia, renal failure, shock.

2. *Chronic pancreatitis*

   Irreversible parenchymal changes.

   Causes: Alcohol, gallstones, idiopathic, CF.

   Features: Abdominal pain, steatorrhoea (malabsorption), weight loss, diabetes.

   Pancreatic calcification on AXR.

How do you manage this condition?

Mary, 27 years on ...

Mary's third problem, which necessitated another visit to the hospital, happened when she was 67 years old. In order to look at this problem we have to turn the clock forward some 20 years. Much has changed in Sunningdale Avenue. Mary is living alone now; Albert, Irene and John having passed away. The children have all left home.

Things didn't work out very well for Mary since John's death some 5 years ago. She regularly suffers from anxiety and bouts of crushing depression. Dr Smith (now 65 and semi-retired), had, on several occasions, suggested counselling and antidepressants but Mary had refused. 'I take a small drink or two every day' – she had not told the whole truth – 'That helps. . .'.

Initially she was brought to see Dr Smith by Matilda, her next-door neighbour, who was worried sick about her. Mary was not eating much and was neglecting herself. She had become more forgetful. Matilda had seen her – through the bay window – wandering around the house in the middle of the night. Matilda's husband, Ivor, found her in the street not too far from her house one night when he was coming back from the pub. Mary could not recognize him at first and appeared confused. He said, 'What are you doing here? It's 11 o'clock. You should be in bed.' She replied, 'I am going to the post office to collect my pension.' He was concerned that she was not dressed properly in the cold night air. He took her home.

On opening the door, Ivor was struck by an unpleasant smell, which reminded him of the filthy public toilet opposite to the derelict bingo hall by the brook. He found a dirty kitchen with a sticky floor and a pile of dirty dishes in the sink. He put the kettle on and washed a cup. He could not find any milk in the fridge. In fact he found an almost empty fridge. When he looked into her food cupboard and her pantry, there was very little food. There was some stale bread and biscuit crumbs on top of the dining table.

He decided to go home and fetch his wife. Matilda felt physically sick when she helped Mary to bed. The bed sheets were stained with dried urine and faeces. She also found at least two dozen empty whisky bottles in her bedroom and sitting room.

She felt angry that Mary's children had not been to see her for such a long time and guilty for not enquiring about Mary's well being. 'I'll make an appointment for you to see Dr Smith tomorrow.' she told Mary.

Dr Smith found her reasonably orientated but her recent memory was not good. She was not as bright as she had been. She appeared cheerful and keen when they were talking about their home football team which Mary supported since she married John who had been a loyal fan.

'I am fine' Mary told him. 'I am only a bit tired and don't feel like eating too much, but I am always like that. I'm just a bit concerned about my tummy. It is embarrassing. I can't button up my skirt. I am not getting fat and definitely not pregnant.'

Dr Smith examined Mary. Her sclerae were mildly yellow and her skin looked dark. Palmar erythema was noted in both hands, and spider naevi were observed on her anterior chest wall. Her abdominal veins were prominent. The spleen was just palpable but the liver was impalpable. He detected ascites. He checked her weight; there was evidence of some weight loss.

Dr Smith suggested to Matilda – who had accompanied Mary to the surgery – to contact Mary's children. He also got permission from Mary to contact Social Services for an assessment.

He ordered some tests, which came back a week later. These are shown in Table 3.2.

What are the mechanisms underlying Mary's signs and symptoms?
Can you interpret the laboratory findings?
What is your preliminary diagnosis?

Mary was jaundiced. The causes of jaundice can be divided into prehepatic, intrahepatic and posthepatic causes.

Table 3.2 Mary's initial investigations

Blood

Bilirubin 210 (0–18 μmol/L)
Unconjugated bilirubin 40 μmol/L
Conjugated bilirubin 170 μmol/L
Total proteins 58 (61–84 g/L)
Albumin 25 (40–52 g/L)
Alkaline phosphatase (Alk Phos.) 155 (0–145 u/L)
Gamma glutamyltransferase (GGT) 225(0–40 u/L)
Aspartate aminotransferase (AST) 110 (5–55 u/L)
Alanine aminotransferase (ALT) 80 (5–55 u/L)
Hb 11.5 (12–16 g/dL)
MCV (mean cell volume) 109 (NR 76–96)
White cell count 13.3 × 10^9/L (4.0–11.0 × 10^9/L)
INR (International Normalized Ratio) 2.6 (NR 1–1.2)

Urine
Bilirubin +
Urobilinogen +.

Serology
Hepatitis A, B and C serology screening: negative

Trigger box **Jaundice**

Raised serum bilirubin.
Detected clinically if >35 μmol/L

1. Prehepatic
   Unconjugated hyperbilirubinaemia.
   Urinary urobilinogen increased. No urine bilirubin.
   Normal liver enzymes.
   Causes
   Overproduction: Haemolysis, reticulocytosis, anaemia.
   Extravascular haemolysis.
   Hereditary spherocytosis.
   Thalassaemia.
   Sickle cell disease.
   G6PD deficiency.
   Autoimmune haemolytic anaemia.
   Intravascular haemolysis.
   Haemolytic transfusion reactions.
   Paroxysmal nocturnal haemoglobinuria.

Impaired conjugation: Reduced UDPGT activity.

Congenital hyperbilirubinaemias (Gilbert's disease, Crigler–Najjar).

Breast milk jaundice.

2. *Hepatic*

Conjugated and unconjugated hyperbilirubinaemia.

Bilirubin present in urine.

Usually AST, ALT, GGT markedly increased; alkaline phosphatase normal or moderately elevated.

Causes

Congenital hyperbilirubinaemias (Dubin–Johnson, Rotor).

Viral hepatitis.

Hepatotoxicity: drugs, chlorinated hydrocarbons (glue sniffing).

Alcoholic disease.

Autoimmune hepatitis.

Haemochromatosis, Wilson's disease.

3. *Posthepatic*

Conjugated hyperbilirubinaemia.

Clinically jaundiced, pale stools (no bile pigments in faeces) and dark urine (increased bile pigments).

Increased urine bilirubin.

Markedly increased alkaline phosphatase, GGT.

Causes

Biliary obstruction.

Gallstones in common bile duct.

Biliary disease.

Pancreatitis.

Carcinoma head of pancreas.

Primary biliary cirrhosis.

Primary sclerosing cholangitis.

The laboratory investigations give us an opportunity to review the functions of the liver. Figure 3.12 shows the formation and circulation of bile salts, an important function of the liver. Note the enterohepatic circulation. Conjugation of bilirubin with glucuronic acid is carried out by UDP-glucuronyl transferase. Deficiencies of this enzyme lead to some key hereditary hyperbilirubinaemias. Other functions of the liver are shown in Table 3.3.

What is the pathology underlying Gilbert's, Rotor, Dubin–Johnson and Crigler–Najjar syndromes?

Over the next two weeks Mary's health deteriorated further. Dr Smith referred her to Hope hospital where further tests were carried out. The results are shown in Table 3.4. She was admitted and started on diuretics (spironolactone and a loop diuretic).

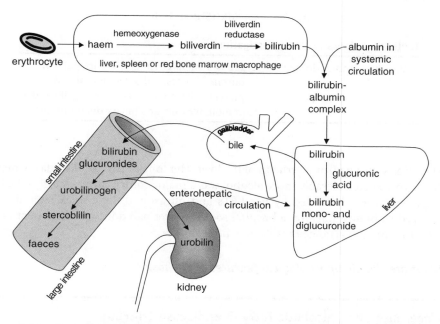

Figure 3.12 Formation and circulation of bile salts. Adapted from Tortora and Grabowski (2003), Principles of Anatomy and Physiology, 10th edition, John Wiley & Sons

Table 3.3 Functions of the liver

Carbohydrate metabolism	Gluconeogenesis Glycogen synthesis Glycogenolysis
Fat metabolism	Cholesterol synthesis Fatty acid synthesis Triglyceride synthesis Ketogenesis Bile and bile acid synthesis
Protein metabolism	Plasma protein synthesis (including some coagulation factors) Urea synthesis
Hormone metabolism	Steroid hormones Peptide hormones
Storage	Glycogen Vitamins A, B_{12} Iron Copper
Detoxification and excretion	Bilirubin Drugs and other foreign compounds Phase 1 detoxification(reduction, oxidation, hydrolysis)involve cytochrome P450 system Phase 2 detoxification involve conjugation (glucoronidation, acetylation)

Table 3.4   Mary's further investigations

Ultrasound scan abdomen	There is a small cirrhotic liver irregular in outline. Ascites and splenomegaly are present. Gallstones seen in the gallbladder. Common bile duct and biliary ducts not dilated

Mary was suffering from cirrhosis of the liver. Her 'one or two drinks a day' which in reality involved considerably more alcohol was a major contributory factor to the liver damage which was indicated by her LFTs and ultrasound. One week later she was discharged from hospital after a hospital social worker had done an assessment of her home situation and arranged meals on wheels for her.

 What are the histopathological features of cirrhosis?

Trigger box   **Non-alcoholic fatty liver disease (NAFLD)**

Caucasians > blacks. Asymptomatic. Exclusion of other chronic liver disease.
Associated with obesity, diabetes, HTN, dyslipidaemia.
Rarely can lead to cirrhosis, hepatocellular carcinoma.
Findings: persistently elevated transaminases (AST/ALT).
Decreased AST:ALT (<1).
'Diffuse increase in echogenicity' on hepatic US.
Treatment: Improves with weight loss, metformin, gemfibrozil, glitazones.

Trigger box   **Alcoholic hepatitis**

May progress to cirrhosis.
Findings: Leukocytosis, Increased MCV & INR, elevated bilirubin, AST, ALT, GGT.
Increased AST:ALT (>1).
Liver biopsy: fatty liver, Mallory bodies.
Treatment: Alcohol abstinence, corticosteroids.

What are Mallory bodies?

Mary's liver damage led to portal hypertension. Figure 3.13 shows the portal system and the important portosystemic anastamosis.

 What are the constituents of bile?

[p = portal, s = systemic]

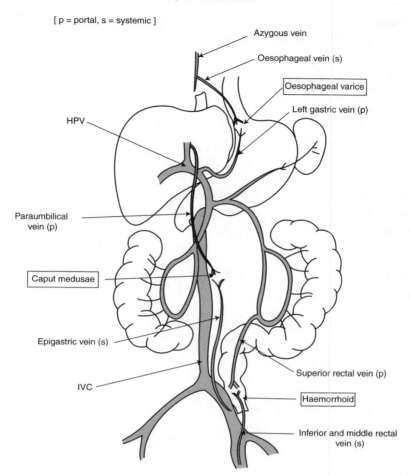

Azygous vein

Oesophageal vein (s)

Oesophageal varice

Left gastric vein (p)

HPV

Paraumbilical
vein (p)

Caput medusae

Epigastric vein (s)

IVC

Superior rectal vein (p)

Haemorrhoid

Inferior and middle rectal
vein (s)

Figure 3.13 Portal-systemic anastamoses

Trigger box Viral hepatitis

Hepatitis A
Acute: IgM for diagnosis.
Faecal–oral transmission
Incubation period (IP):30 days.
Infectious before jaundice.
Moderate hepatomegaly.
Fulminant hepatitis rare.
No chronicity.
Active immunization available.

Hepatitis B

Vertical transmission (most common), IVDA, sex.

IP = 1–5 months.

HbcAb IgM = acute infection.

HbeAg = viral replication/infectivity.

HbsAb = immunity.

HbsAg = carrier state.

HbeAb = low transmissibility.

1% develop fulminant disease.

3% progress to chronic hepatitis.

Chronic carriers inversely related to age of infection.

Risk of cirrhosis and cancer.

Treatment: Interferon-α and/or lamuvidine.

Vaccine available.

Hepatitis C

Blood.

IP = 2–4 months.

Most progress to chronic disease.

Cirrhosis and hepatocellular carcinoma.

Treatment: Interferon-α and ribavirin.

Hepatitis D

Incomplete virus activated by HepB.

IVDA transmission

IgM.

Hepatitis E

Enteral/waterborne transmission.

No chronic carrier state.

Fulminant hepatitis.

Pregnancy.

Mary's ultrasound also showed that she has asymptomatic cholelithiasis. Mary's gall-stones could, if they moved into and obstruct the common bile duct, cause problems of fat digestion and absorption. The failure to excrete bilirubin would lead to conjugated hyperbilirubinaemia (obstructive jaundice) and the inability to secrete bile, essential for fat digestion, would cause steatorrhoea.

 What are the main risk factors for cholelithiasis?

Trigger box   Cholecystitis

Fat, Female, forties, fertile, flatulent.
OCP use, rapid weight loss, chronic haemolysis.

1. *Acute cholecystitis*
   Stone in cystic duct/neck of gall bladder.
   Severe postprandial RUQ pain, fever, tenderness, guarding.
   Murphy's sign.
   Complications: Empyema, perforation, peritonitis.
   US diagnosis, HIDA scan.
   Treatment: Cefotaxime, cholecystectomy.

2. *Chronic cholecystitis*
   Chronic inflammation due to gallstones.
   Treatment: Cholecystectomy if symptomatic.

What is choledocholithiasis?

 Review the blood supply to the liver.

'Why does everything I eat turn to fat?'

Let us now turn the clock back to the present. We are back in the living room at No 10 Sunningdale Avenue. John and Mary are watching TV and the children are upstairs. Debbie is in her room reading a magazine. She is not happy. She had just weighed herself and was shocked to find that her latest diet had made her put on two pounds! Mary isn't the only one in the house concerned about matters pertaining to digestion. Debbie is obsessed about losing weight and has been on many diets.

This leads us to consider the section of the gastrointestinal tract distal to the duodenum; the small intestine consisting of the jejunum and the ileum and beyond that, the colon and the rectum.

Figure 3.14 shows the main events taking place in the small intestine. Note the key enzymes in pancreatic juice, the key role of enterokinase and the actions of the brush border enzymes.

Table 3.5 shows some key factors involved in digestion.

 Complete Table 3.5.

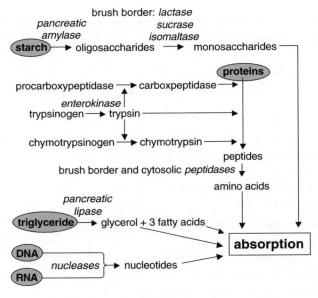

Figure 3.14   Digestion in the small intestine

Trigger Box: Malabsorption

Symptoms	Steatorrhoea: frequent pale, foul-smelling, loose stools Also abdominal pain, flatulence, failure to thrive, weight loss, bloating.
Nutritional deficiencies	Skin and mucosal lesions (trace elements & vitamins), anaemia (iron, folate, vitamin B_{12}), osteomalacia (vitamin D), Bleeding tendencies (vitamin K), peripheral neuropathy (vitamin B_{12}), oedema (hypoproteinaemia).
Causes	Gluten sensitive enteropathies: coeliac disease. Inflammatory bowel disease: Crohn's disease. Pancreatic insufficiency: Chronic pancreatitis, cystic fibrosis. Carbohydrate malabsorption: Lactose intolerance Infection: amoebiasis, giardiasis, *Clostridium difficile*, HIV. Infiltrative bowel disease: Whipple's disease, amyloidosis. Short bowel syndrome: previous surgery.
Treatment	Aetiology dependent: TPN, immunosuppressants Correction of nutritional deficiencies.

Table 3.5 Some factors involved in digestion (complete the table)

Substance	Source	Function	Factors regulating secretion
Cholecystokinin			Fatty acids, amino acids
Somatostatin			
Secretin	Duodenum (S cell)		
Vasoactive intestinal peptide			

Absorption is shown in Figure 3.15.

 Describe the blood supply to the small and large intestine. What is the watershed area?

What is the pathophysiology of coeliac disease?

Acute gastroenteritis with diarrhoea and vomiting is a common GI complaint. It maybe infective (shigellosis, salmonellosis, *E. coli*, cholera toxin) or non-infective and usually resolve within 4 weeks. Chronic diarrhoea is diarrhoea persisting for over 4 weeks.

Trigger box Chronic diarrhoea

Passage of loose or liquid stools more than three times a day and/or stool weight >200 g/day.

1. *Osmotic diarrhoea*: Stool osmotic gap >125 mOsm/kg.
   Causes: laxatives, malabsorption defect (e.g. disaccharidase deficiency), stops when feeding stops.

2. *Secretory diarrhoea*: Stool osmotic gap,< 50 mOsm/kg.
   Causes: Colon cancer, coeliac disease, drugs and food additives, inflammatory bowel disease, chronic infection (amoebiasis, giardiais, HIV, bacterial overgrowth), neuroendocrine tumours (VIPomas, gastrinomas, carcinoid), villous adenoma.
   Continues when fasting.

3. *Motility-related diarrhoea*:
   Causes: Thyrotoxicosis, diabetic autonomic neuropathy, post vagotomy.

4. *Functional diarrhoea*:
   Irritable bowel syndrome (IBS).

   Investigations:

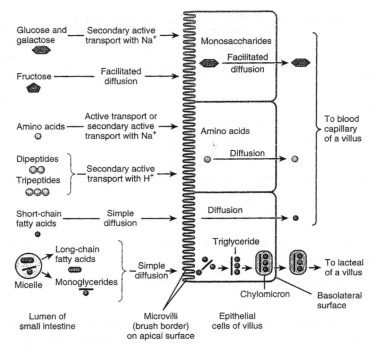

(a) Mechanisms for movement of nutrients through absorptive epithelial cells of the villi

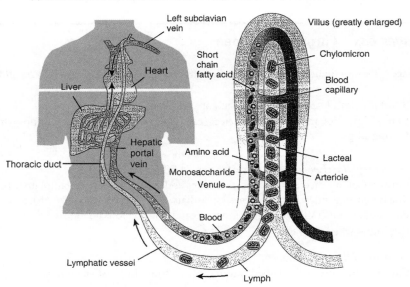

(b) Movement of absorbed nutrients into the blood and lymph

Figure 3.15   Absorption of digested nutrients in the small intestine (N.B. some are digested by brush-border enzymes). Adapted from Tortora and Grabowski (2003), Principles of Anatomy and Physiology, 10th Edition, John Wiley and Sons Inc. New York

Measure 24 hr stool weight

Stool osmotic gap $\{290 - 2 (Na^+ + K^+)\}$

Coeliac serology, hydrogen breath tests for bacterial overgrowth or carbohydrate intolerance, stool culture/ microscopy, barium studies, faecal elastase/chymotrypsin, CT, ERCP, MRCP.

Sigmoidoscopy, colonoscopy and biopsy, barium enema.

Laxative screen, serum gastrin, serum VIP, and urine 5HIAA.

How would you treat these different types of diarrhoeal illnesses?

Trigger box **Key diarrhoeal infections**

Campylobacter jejuni

Most common diarrhoeal pathogen

Can cause septicaemia

Food/water borne infection, poultry

IP = 2–7days

Lasts 9 days

Faecal WBC/RBC, rods on microscopy

Erythromycin.

Escherichia coli 0157; H7

Transmission: raw meat, milk

IP = 12–48 h

Bloody diarrhoea, severe abdominal pain, fever, vomiting, faecal WBC/RBC

Children/elderly more susceptible

Lasts 8 days

No antibiotics.

Salmonella

Poultry/eggs transmission

Sepsis possible

Children/elderly more susceptible

IP = 24 h

Lasts 5 days

Headache, fever, abdominal pain, faecal WBC/RBC

5–10% become bacteraemic.

Shigella

Faecal–oral transmission

Toxin

IP = 48 h

Children/institutionalized more susceptible

Bloody mucoid diarrhoea, faecal WBC/RBC, febrile seizures, dehydration

Ciprofloxacin.

Clostridium difficile

Pathology: pseudomembanous colitis

Clindamycin use

Fever, abdominal pain, faecal WBC, RBC, *C. difficile* toxin in stool

Tx metronidazole/vancomycin

Complication: toxic megacolon.

Entamoeba histolytica

Food/water transmission, travel related, sexual transmission

Severe abdominal pain, faecal WBC/RBC, colitis

IP variable

Bloody diarrhoea, colitic, toxic dilatation, perforation, peritonitis, liver abscess, flask like ulcers

Fluorescent antibody test, cysts

Metronidazole, dolixanide furoate.

Trigger box   Inflammatory bowel disease

1. *Ulcerative colitis*
   1:1000.

   Age range:20–40 years.

   Episodic bloody diarrhoea often with mucus. Weight loss, fever, anaemia.

   Extra-intestinal manifestations: Erythema nodosum, pyoderma gangrenosum, clubbing, arthritis, hepatitis, cirrhosis, cholangitis, iritis, episcleritis.

   Only colon affected. Rectum then proximal extension.

   Mucosal inflammation, continuous lesions, ulcers and pseudopolyps, crypt abscesses.

   Bowel complication: Toxic megalcolon.

   Cancer risk.

   Treatment: 5-ASA compounds (e.g. mesalamine), corticosteroids, immunosuppressives (e.g. azothiaprine), surgery.

2. *Crohn's disease*
   Mouth to anus: commonest ileocaecal.

   Abdominal pain and distension, bloody diarrhoea, weight loss, fever, anaemia, malabsorption.

   Extra-intestinal manifestations: Erythema nodusum, pyoderma gangrenosum, clubbing, arthritis, hepatitis, cirrhosis, cholangitis, iritis.

   Skip lesions, cobblestone mucosa, string sign (fibrosis),

   Transmural inflammation, non-caesating granulomata, abscesses, fibrosis.

   Bowel complications: Stricture, obstruction, fistula, perforation.

   Treatment: 5-ASA compounds (e.g. mesalamine), corticosteroids, immunosuppressives (e.g. azothiaprine), anti-tumour necrosis factor-α, (anti-TNF α) metronidazole, surgery.

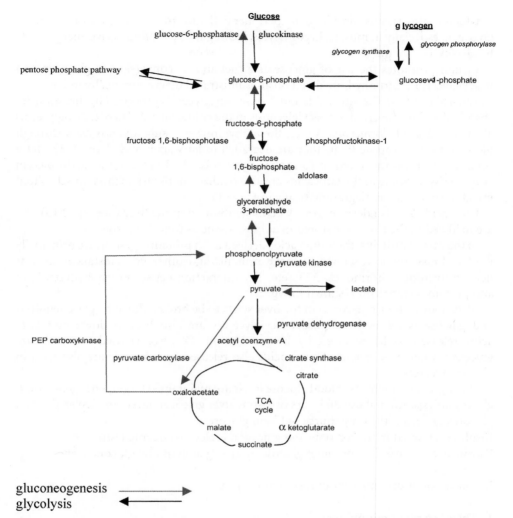

Figure 3.16 Carbohydrate metabolism. Adapted from Stryer (1988), Biochemistry, 3rd edition, Freeman

Debbie decided to try another new diet. She had been reading about a new diet, which severely reduced carbohydrate intake. Debbie's concerns lead us to consider what happens to the absorbed nutrients. This involves understanding the principles of carbohydrate, lipid and protein catabolism and anabolism. We will cover carbohydrate and lipid metabolism in this chapter. Protein metabolism will be considered in more depth in Chapter 4. Cholesterol metabolism was considered in Chapter 2.

Let us start with carbohydrates. After a meal glucose enters the liver via the hepatic portal vein. Some of this glucose is oxidized to meet the immediate energy needs and the remainder is converted to glycogen or triacylglycerols and stored.

Glucose also travels via blood to peripheral tissues to be oxidized or stored as glycogen, especially in muscle. Erythrocytes, lacking mitochondria derive energy solely by glycolysis.

Insulin promotes the use of glucose as a fuel and its conversion to glycogen and triacylglycerols. Carbohydrate metabolism is illustrated diagrammatically in Fig. 3.16.

What about fats? The fatty acids and 2-monoacylglycerols produced by digestion are absorbed and reconverted to triacylglycerols in the epithelial cell. These triacylglycerols are released as chylomicrons. When these chylomicrons subsequently pass through blood vessels in adipose tissue they are degraded to fatty acids and glycerol. The fatty acids recombine with glycerol to form triacylglycerols, which are stored as fat droplets in adipose tissue. Some of the fatty acids are also oxidized in tissues such as muscle. Lipid metabolism is shown diagrammatically in Fig. 3.17.

Fatty acids are also derived from VLDLs synthesised in the liver (See Fig. 2.15) and are oxidized in the tissues or stored in adipose tissue as triacylglycerols.

In the case of proteins, the amino acids derived from protein digestion are principally used in biosynthetic reactions to make proteins and other key substances such as neurotransmitters, hormones, ATP, etc. The interaction between carbohydrate, lipid and protein metabolism is shown in Fig. 3.18.

After about 3 hours glycogen in the liver starts to be broken down by glycogenolysis and glucose is released. Adipose triacylglycerols are also broken down and fatty acids released to be oxidized by beta oxidation. Glycerol is used to synthesize glucose via gluconeogenesis. Amino acids also released from muscle are also used in gluconeogenesis.

During an overnight fast blood glucose levels are maintained by gluconeogenesis and glycogenolysis. After about 30 hours of fasting liver glycogen levels are depleted. Then gluconeogenesis is the only source of blood glucose.

Insulin is elevated in the fed state and glucagon is elevated during fasting.

During exercise the liver provides glucose by glycogenolysis and gluconeogenesis.

Key facts you must know about these pathways are:

1. Their key rate-limiting steps

2. The enzymes involved in these steps, and,

3. The factors that regulate these key enzymes, especially (where relevant) the roles of insulin, glucagon epinephrine and cortisol.

Carefully complete Table 3.6: very useful for revision!!

Construct a diagram showing the metabolic changes seen in the fed, fasting and starvation states.

What are the functions of the large intestine?

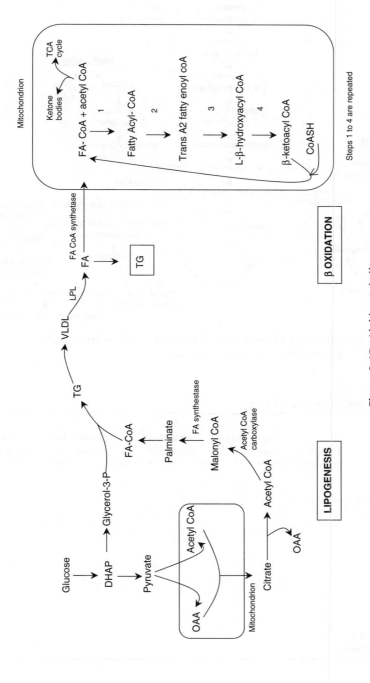

Figure 3.17 Lipid metabolism

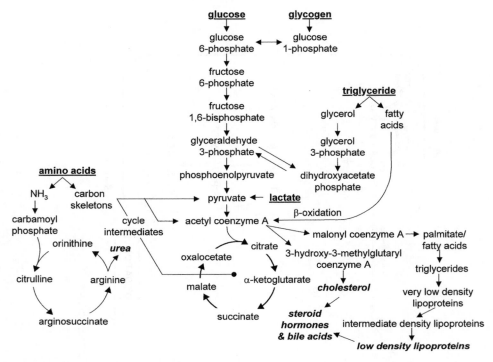

Figure 3.18   Interrelationship between carbohydrate, lipid and protein metabolism. Adapted from Stryer (1988), *Biochemistry, 3rd edition, Freeman*

Table 3.6   Key features of metabolism

Metabolic pathway	Location	Key regulatory enzymes	Key regulatory metabolites	Hormonal controls	Clinical significance
Glycolysis					
Glycogenolysis					
Pentose phosphate pathway					
Gluconeogenesis					
Glycogenesis					
Lipogenesis					
Beta oxidation					
Ketogenesis					
TCA cycle					
Ketone body metabolism					
Ethanol metabolism					
Cholesterol synthesis					

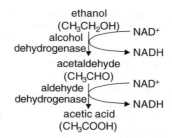

Figure 3.19 Ethanol metabolism. Adapted from Stryer (1988), Biochemistry, 3rd edition, Freeman

We can finish this section by briefly looking at Mary's alcohol problem and then consider vitamins and minerals. Alcohol metabolism is shown in Figure 3.19.

Mary always maintained that alcohol wasn't a drug and that she wasn't a drug addict. Figure 3.20 shows the pharmacokinetics of alcohol which shows zero kinetics. Figure 3.20 also shows the kinetics of a first order drug elimination.

Mary's alcohol problems could have led to a thiamin deficiency. Debbie's dieting could also cause vitamin and mineral deficiency. Functions and deficiencies associated with vitamins and key minerals are shown in Table 3.7.

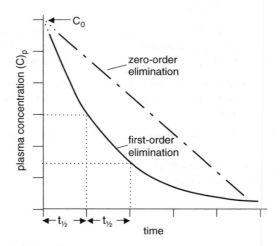

Figure 3.20 Zero and first order kinetics ($t\frac{1}{2}$ = half-life, C_0 = apparent initial plasma concentration). For first-order elimination rate of elimination is proportional to concentration. For zero-order kinetics the rate of elimination occurs at a constant rate

Table 3.7   Functions and deficiencies associated with key vitamins and minerals

	Functions	Major clinical features of deficiency
Fat-soluble vitamins		
A (retinol)	Constituent of retinol Growths & differentiation of epithelia and bone. Gametogenesis, vision	Xerophthalmia, night blindness, keratomalacia Follicular hyperkeratosis.
D (cholecalciferol)	Increases gut absorption of calcium & phosphate Mineralization of bone matrix (osteoid)	Rickets in children. Osteomalacia in adults. Vague bone and muscle pain.
K	Production of blood clotting factors (carboxylation of Glu residues) Formation of bone by osteoblasts	Coagulation defects. Vit K dep factors: II, VII, IX, X, protein C and S.
E (α-tocopherol)	Antioxidant Membrane stability	In young children neurological disorders, e.g. ataxia.
Water-soluble vitamins		
B_1 (thiamin)	Carbohydrate metabolism Coenzyme in oxidative decarboxylation of α keto acids and required in the HMP shunt	Beriberi (polyneuropathy), Wernicke–Korsakoff syndrome (cerebral involvement).
B_2 (riboflavin)	Cofactor in carbohydrate and lipid metabolism (e.g. FAD, FMN)	Angular stomatitis, red inflamed tongue, seborrhoeic dermatitis.
Niacin B3	Oxidative and reductive reactions (active part in NAD^+ & $NADPH^+$)	Pellagra (dermatitis, diarrhoea, dementia).
B_6 (pyridoxine)	Metabolism of several amino acids (e.g. in transamination) Neurotransmitter synthesis.	Polyneuropathy.

Table 3.7 (*Continued*)

	Functions	Major clinical features of deficiency
B_{12} (cobalamin)	Cofactor for homocysteine methylation. Isomerization of methylmalonyl CoA to succinyl CoA: synthesis of bases in DNA and RNA.	Megaloblastic anaemia, Neurological disorders
Folate	Cofactor for homocysteine methylation. One carbon addition reactions: synthesis of bases in DNA and RNA.	Megaloblastic anaemia
C (ascorbic acid)	Redox potential within cells. Formation of collagen, Fe absorption	Scurvy
Minerals		
Iron	Constituent of haemoglobin	Anaemia
Copper	In a variety of enzymes	Menkes' kinky hair syndrome
Zinc	In a variety of enzymes	Acrodermatitis enteropathica, impaired wound healing, impaired taste & smell, hair loss, night blindness
Iodine	Constituent of thyroid hormones	'Endemic goitre'
Selenium	Preventing oxidative and free radical damage to cells	Selenium-responsive cardiomyopathy
Calcium	Mineral salts of the bone and teeth Intracellular function eg contraction of muscles	Osteoporosis

 Find out about the functions and deficiency diseases associated with biotin.

4

The urinary system

Learning strategy

The urinary system is basically a filtration system, whose main function is to remove waste products from the body and maintain homeostasis.

A good way to learn the key facts and concepts of the urinary system is to consider the different parts of the process leading to the formation of urine: filtration, reabsorption and secretion. Reabsorption and secretion, which is carried out by the kidney tubules also allows us to consider other homeostatic functions of the kidney such as regulation of acid–base, electrolytes and blood pressure. Our discussion will also briefly consider the endocrine functions of the kidney.

The storyline attempts to illustrate these major facts and concepts by considering clinical scenarios involving renal dysfunction caused by prerenal, intrinsic renal and postrenal factors.

As you read these scenarios, it is important to review the normal anatomy, embryology, and physiology of the renal system in addition to understanding the pathophysiological basis of the disease processes. Also reviewing the mechanisms of action of the key diuretics will help reinforce functions of the different segments of the kidney tubules.

Try to answer the questions and try to complete the Learning Tasks.

Integrated Medical Sciences   by Shantha Perera, Stephen Anderson, Ho Leung and Rousseau Gama
© 2007 John Wiley & Sons, Ltd   ISBN: 978470016589 (HB) 978470016596 (PB)

Max's great pain

Max woke up one night suffering from excruciating left-sided loin pain, which was radiating to his left testis. Debbie, who was staying with him at the time, immediately rang 999. The paramedics found the young man writhing in his bed. He was sweating, pale and complained of feeling nauseous. Max was in agony; it was the most severe pain he had ever experienced. The paramedics gave him morphine and rushed him to the Emergency Department at Hope hospital.

One of the physicians checked him out. Max's pulse was 115 per min, respiratory rate 23 per min, BP 168/91 and he was febrile with a temperature of 38 °C. Abdominal examination revealed left loin tenderness and pain on palpation. There were no masses.

Urinalysis found blood, but no protein and casts. A full blood count revealed leukocytosis (13×10^9/L). A plain abdominal X-ray showed a 2 mm faint calcified lesion in the left hemipelvis. Ultrasound indicated a calculus in the lower end of left ureter with proximal dilatation of the ureter and renal pelvis.

Max was given more morphine. Within half-hour his pain was better but he had to have more analgesia later. The doctor informed Max that if he did not pass the stone spontaneously he might have to undergo surgery for removal of the stone.

How are kidney stones formed? Where are they most likely to be found

Check out the Trigger box on nephrolithiasis.

Trigger box   **Nephrolithiasis**

Males > female.

Usually over the age of 40 years.

Composition: Calcium oxalate (85%), magnesium ammonium phosphate ('infection' or 'struvite' stones), uric acid (hyperuricosuria), cystine (cystinuria).

Risk factors: Low fluid intake, family history, diet (oxalate, e.g. in spinach; uric acid e.g. animal protein), infection (urease producing organisms, e.g. *Proteus, Klebsiella*), diseases (idiopathic hypercalciuria, gout, renal tubular acidosis (RTA), primary hyperparathyroidism).

Features: Severe colic, pain radiates to testes/vulva.

Findings: Microscopic or frank haematuria, proteinuria.

Radio-opaque – calcium, magnesium ammonium phosphate, cysteine.

Radiolucent – uric acid, xanthine.

Investigations: IVP, serum calcium and uric acid, urine cysteine, 24 hour urine calcium, oxalate and urate.

Treatment: Hydration, analgesia, extracorporeal shock wave lithotripsy, percutaneous nephrolithotomy, endoscopic stone removal.

Treat underlying cause.

Prevention: High fluid intake and appropriate diet.

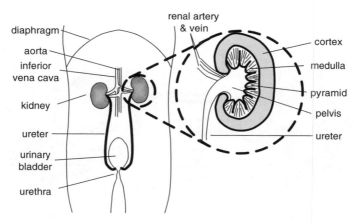

Figure 4.1 Gross anatomy of the urinary system. Adapted from Tortoa and Grabowski (2003), Principles of Anatomy and Physiology, 10th edition, John Wiley & Sons

Max's problem leads us to consider the gross anatomy of the urinogenital system. Figure 4.1 shows the gross anatomy of the urinogenital organs. Note the two kidneys, the main blood vessels and ureters, the bladder and the urethra.

Where are the kidneys located? Where are they relative to other abdominal structures?
The kidneys are retroperitoneal organs. What does this mean? What other organs are retroperitoneal?

 Draw a diagram illustrating the fasciae surrounding the kidney

Max's brother Peter had died a few days after birth. Peter had suffered from oligohydramnios where the volume of amniotic fluid was less than normal. This was due a rare case of bilateral renal agenesis where the ureteric bud had degenerated early, failing to reach the metanephros.

What is the metanephros? What is the ureteric bud?

We have to consider the development of the urinary system in order to understand these terms. The embryology of the renal system is linked to that of the genital system. The latter will be considered in Chapter 8. Here we will focus on the embryology of the urinary system, which is illustrated in Figure 4 2.

The urinary system develops from mesoderm. The development of the mature urinary system involves the successive formation of three kidney systems: a pronephros, a mesonephros and finally a metanephros which appears in the 5th week. The pronephros and mesonephros disappear to give way to the kidney proper.

The ureters, calcyes, renal pelves, and the collecting system develop from an ureteric bud, an outgrowth of the mesonephric duct, as seen in Figure 4.2. Early division of the ureteric bud can lead to supernumerary kidneys with ectopic ureters. If the ureteric bud

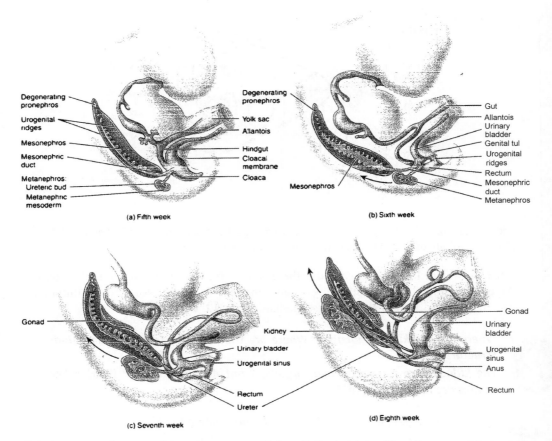

Figure 4.2 lists labels:

(a) Fifth week — Degenerating pronephros, Urogenital ridges, Mesonephros, Mesonephric duct, Metanephros: Ureteric bud, Metanephric mesoderm; Degenerating pronephros, Yolk sac, Allantois, Hindgut, Cloacal membrane, Cloaca

(b) Sixth week — Gut, Allantois, Urinary bladder, Genital tul, Urogenital ridges, Rectum, Mesonephric duct, Metanephros, Mesonephros

(c) Seventh week — Gonad, Kidney, Urinary bladder, Urogenital sinus, Rectum, Ureter

(d) Eighth week — Gonad, Urinary bladder, Urogenital sinus, Anus, Rectum

Figure 4.2 Development of the urinary system (full credit line). Adapted from Tortora and Grabowski (2003), Principles of Anatomy and Physiology, 10th Edition, John Wiley and Sons Inc. New York

fails to form this can cause renal agenesis. Failure of the ureteric bud to branch can lead to the failure of formation of the collecting tubes.

The kidney is initially found in the pelvic region but later ascends upward. The blood supply thus changes from pelvic branches of the aorta to branches derived from higher levels of the great vessel.

Supernumerary renal arteries may result from persistence of embryonic vessels. Other abnormalities include pelvic kidneys and horseshoe kidneys.

By the third month the fetal kidneys begin to excrete urine. Urine passes into the amniotic cavity and mixes with the amniotic fluid, which is swallowed by the fetus. This fluid is then reabsorbed and passed through the kidneys back into the amniotic fluid.

What is horseshoe kidney? What happens to this structure during the 'ascent' of the kidney?

What are the underlying mechanisms leading to the amniotic fluid anomalies, polyhydramnios and oligohydramnios?

> ### *Trigger box* Polycystic kidney disease
>
> AD variety most common.
>
> Presents between age 20–50 years, usually with end-stage renal failure.
>
> 50% will have a family history.
>
> **Features:** Pain, haematuria, palpable kidneys, hypertension (HTN) liver cysts, berry aneurysms, mitral valve prolapse.
>
> US/CT for diagnosis.
>
> **Treatment:** BP control, dialysis and renal transplant in end-stage disease.
>
> AR variety is rare but of greater severity. More common in children and infants and may present in utero.

Max is fighting, and losing...again!

Two months later, Max went missing. Debbie had last seen him at their local pub on Friday night. Max had appeared restless, quieter than usual, but on questioning had not revealed any particular problems or worries. Debbie knew better; she had seen Max like this before; it had always meant problems. But he was reticent and Debbie knew better than to push him. He had walked her home and had promised to call her early next day. By Saturday evening Debbie had begun to get worried: she hadn't heard from him; and his mobile appeared to be switched off.

Late Saturday evening Debbie received a call from the hospital. Max had been found lying in a field on the outskirts of town by some walkers who had immediately called the paramedics. Max appeared to have received a severe beating. When the paramedics found him he was dehydrated and his BP was 95/70 with a heart rate of 120/min. His core body temp was 36 °C. In the ambulance Max was given oxygen, i.v. fluids and morphine. He began complaining of severe pain all over his body. He was rushed to the ED.

 What does the low BP reading suggest?

At the ED the attending physician found Max confused and disorientated with periods of lucidity. There were no broken bones and no obvious cervical spine or head trauma. His mucous membranes were dry and his skin was flaccid, lacking normal turgor. His abdomen was tender but without guarding or rebound. Max's cardiovascular and respiratory examination was normal except for a tachycardia (115/min) and a respiratory rate of 28/min. His neurological examination was also normal with no focal neurological signs. The doctor suspected that Max's main problem was internal abdominal bleeding.

Max was also oliguric. Max's oliguria indicates that his injuries have affected his renal function. This allows us to begin our exploration of the functioning of the renal system. Figure 4.3 shows the nephron, the filtration unit of the kidney. Note the afferent and

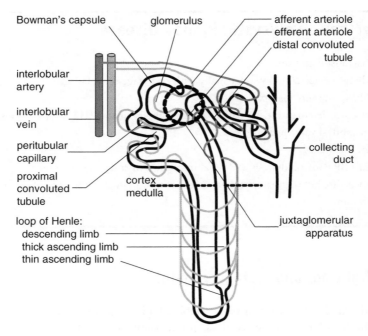

Figure 4.3 Nephron ultrastructure

efferent arterioles, the glomerulus and Bowman's capsule, the tubular organization and the peritubular blood supply.

Table 4.1 outlines the main functions of the kidney.

Max was in acute renal failure brought about by a greatly reduced blood supply to these vital organs. The lack of blood supply was most likely due to the internal haemorrhage suffered as a consequence of his beating. Additionally his dehydration contributed to his low volume status. As 25 per cent of the cardiac output flows through the kidneys, a drop in Max's renal blood flow led to a decrease in the hydrostatic pressure in the glomerulus. This led to a decrease in glomerular filtration and reduced urine output. Figure 4.4 shows the main forces acting at the glomerulus involved in filtration.

Table 4.1 Main kidney functions

Glomerular function	Excretion of toxic end-products of metabolism and foreign substances.
Tubular function	Acid–base, water and electrolyte balance.
Endocrine function	1,25 dihydroxycholecalciferol: calcium metabolism. Erythropoietin: haemoglobin synthesis.
	Renin (renin–angiotensin–aldosterone system): salt and electrolyte balance.
Carbohydrate metabolism	Gluconeogenesis.

Which plasma component contributes to plasma oncotic pressure?

Trigger box   Acute renal failure

Characterized by oliguria (<300 ml/day) or anuria.

Metabolic acidosis (inability to excrete H^+ ions).

Hyperkalaemia (due to decreased renal excretion and acidosis).

Pulmonary oedema due to salt and water retention (often iatrogenic).

Rising serum urea and creatinine.

In early stages features depends on underlying cause. In later stages malaise, anorexia, nausea, vomiting, pericarditis (pericardial rub), encephalopathy (asterixis, confusion, convulsions, coma).

Types:

1. **Prerenal**

   Causes: Hypovolaemia (haemorrhage, dehydration, burns), cardiogenic shock, septicaemic shock, drugs (NSAIDs), renal artery stenosis.

   Can lead to orthostasis and hypotension.

2. **Intrinsic renal**

   Causes: Intrinsic renal parenchymal disease (acute tubular necrosis, acute glomerulonephritis), collagen vascular diseases (polyarteritis nodosa, systemic lupus erythematosus), haemolytic uraemic syndrome, drugs (aminoglycosides), metabolic (diabetes), sepsis (e.g. surgical sepsis), thromboembolism.

3. **Postrenal**

   Urinary obstruction.

   Causes: Prostate disease, kidney stones, pelvic and retroperitoneal tumours and fibrosis.

   Distended bladder if bladder outflow obstructed.

   Treatment

   Prerenal: Rapid correction of hypovolaemia. Fluid/electrolyte balance.

   Intrinsic renal: Steroids, immunosuppressants.

   Postrenal: Prompt relief of obstruction.

   Indications for dialysis: Hyperkalaemia, pulmonary oedema, acidosis, uraemia.

   Emergencies:

   Hyperkalaemia: intravenous calcium (cardioprotection), intravenous dextrose and insulin (lowers plasma potassium), dialysis.

   Pulmonary oedema: diuretics, dialysis.

List the main features of chronic renal failure.

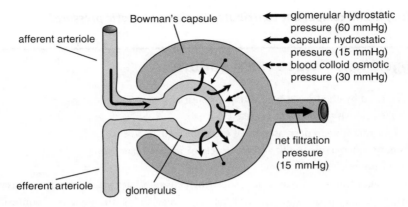

Figure 4.4 Forces acting at the glomerular capillary. Adapted form Tortora and Grabowski (2003), Principles of Anatomy and Physiology, 10th edition, John Wiley & Sons

Max was also dehydrated, and, in an attempt to conserve water more tubular reabsorption was also taking place. This contributed to his oliguria. The physician ordered a battery of tests; the results are shown in Table 4.2.

Table 4.2 Laboratory findings

Haematology	FBC Hb: 9.2 g/dL WCC: 17.6× 10^9/L, platelets: normal; ESR 31 mm/h
Biochemistry	Na^+: 142 mmol/L (135–145 mmol/L)
	K^+: 6.5 mmol/L (3.5–5.0 mmol/L)
	Urea: 21.6 mmol/L(2.1–9.0 mmol/L)
	Creatinine: 0.77 mmol/L (0.06–0.13 mmol/L)
	Calcium: 2.11 mmol/L (2.10–2.60 mmol/L)
	Phosphate: 2.86 mmol/L (0.8–0.14 mmol/L)
	Bicarbonate: 13 mmol/L (22–25 mmol/L)
	Creatine kinase: 124 000 IU/L (<150 IU/L)
	Bilirubin: 40 µmol/L (1–18 µmol/L)
	AST: 450 IU/L (5–40 IU/L) ALT: 124 IU/L (5–40 IU/L)
	Cl^-, total protein and albumin all normal
ECG	Tall peaked T waves, broad QRS complex
Urine microscopy	1200 RBC/mL, 250 WBC/mL, numerous granular casts seen
Urine biochemistry	Urine electrolytes: Na^+ 55 mmol/L; K^+ 52 mmol/L
Urine osmolality	290 mOsm/kg
Urinary myoglobin	Positive
Arterial blood gases	pH 7.26 (7.38–7.44)
	PaO_2 14.0 KPa (9–13 KPa)
	$PaCO_2$ 3.0 KPa (4–6 KPa)
	HCO_3^- 10 mmol/L (22–25)
Radiology	Renal ultrasound – normal
	X-rays – right hip, left hip, pelvis – all normal.

What is the significance of the raised CPK?
Why were the AST and ALT raised?

 Describe the different types of urinary casts indicating their clinical significance.

Let us consider some of these results, as they will allow us to delve more deeply into what is going on in the glomerulus. Let us look at the urea and creatinine results first. Max has increased urea and creatinine. This means that the most important function of the kidneys, the elimination of metabolic waste products has been compromised. Figure 4.5 shows nitrogen metabolism and the urea cycle.

 What are the principal excretory products eliminated via the kidneys?

Why have Max's urea and creatinine levels increased? Plasma creatinine is produced at a steady rate by muscle creatine breakdown and eliminated via the kidneys. Plasma creatinine levels are inversely proportional to the glomerular filtration rate (GFR). So Max's increased creatinine levels indicated a drop in the GFR, which in turn was initially caused by reduced renal blood flow (RBF) which if prolonged may also lead to acute tubular necrosis. Tubular deposition of myoglobin may also be a contributing factor. However, as seen in Figure 4.6 the GFR must be reduced by around 50 per cent before a significant increase in creatinine levels is seen.

The GFR is a good index of renal glomerular function. The GFR can be estimated by measuring the clearance of a substance that is neither reabsorbed nor secreted by the kidney tubules. Clinically, creatinine clearance is used as only a non-significant amount of creatinine is secreted and none is reabsorbed by the renal tubules. Plasma creatinine is therefore a convenient albeit insensitive marker of GFR.

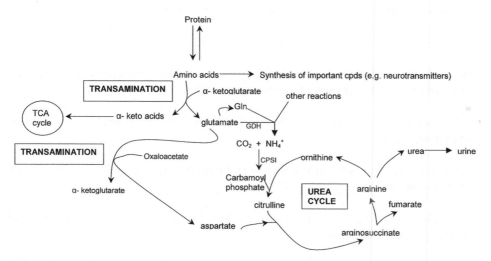

Figure 4.5 Protein metabolism. GDH = glutamate dehydrogenase, CPSI = carbamoyl phosphate synthetase I. Adapted from Marks et al (1996). *Basic Medical Biochemistry. William & Wilkins*

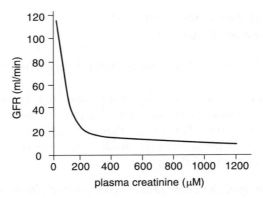

Figure 4.6   Relationship between plasma creatinine and GFR. Adapted from Boron and Boulpaep (2003), Medical Physiology, Saunders

The concept of clearance is very relevant to renal function. Clearance refers to the virtual volume of plasma cleared of a substance in a given time. Clearance is, therefore, affected by glomerular filtration, tubular reabsorption and tubular secretion.

You need to understand clearance equations!

$$\text{Clearance of substance } Z = U \times V/P$$

Where U = concentration of Z in urine, V = volume collected in a given period of time and P = concentration of Z in plasma.

So how can we calculate the glomerular filtration rate (GFR)? The GFR can be calculated by applying the clearance equation to creatinine

$$\text{GFR} = U \times V/P$$

Where U = concentration of creatinine in urine, V = volume collected in a given period of time and P = concentration of creatinine in plasma.

- If the clearance for a substance is greater than GFR then there is net tubular secretion of that substance

- If the clearance for a substance is less than GFR then there is net tubular reabsorption of that substance

- If the clearance for a substance is same as GFR then there is no tubular secretion or reabsorption of that substance.

Renal plasma flow (RPF) can be estimated by measuring the clearance of a substance that is totally removed from the blood in a single circuit through the kidneys. This requires filtration and secretion of the substance (for example *para*-aminohippuric acid, PAH) such that none remains in the outgoing renal vein. PAH is used to measure RPF.

$$RPF = U \times V/P$$

Where U = concentration of PAH in urine, V = volume collected in a given period of time and P = concentration of PAH in plasma.

The filtration fraction is the fraction of renal plasma that is filtered through the glomeruli and it can be calculated from the above formulae.

$$\text{Filtration fraction (FF)} = GFR/RBF$$

If the RPF = 650 ml/min, assuming a haematocrit of 45 per cent, calculate the renal blood flow (RBF).

Max's cola urine

Max was no stranger to kidney problems. When he was 8 years old he suffered from another kidney condition, post-streptococcal glomerulonephritis (PSGN). Let's look at what happened.

Max suffered from a sore throat, which resolved after 5 days. However, some 2 weeks later, he presented to his GP with facial swelling and reduced urine output with the urine having a pinkish colour. The GP noted periorbital and ankle oedema. Max's BP was 132/ 93. He was referred to a paediatrician at the local hospital.

At the hospital Max was found to have mild anaemia, proteinuria, hypoalbuminae-mia, hyperkalaemia and low C3 levels. Tests also indicated abnormal kidney function with raised urea and creatinine. MSU analysis showed numerous erythrocytes and granular casts but no growth. A throat swab culture was negative. The paediatrician then requested an ASO titre, which came up positive. As the clinical diagnosis of PSGN following a Lancefield group A β-haemolytic streptococcus infection was clear-cut, he did not order a renal biopsy or a renal imaging.

If a renal biopsy was carried out what would have been found?

Max was treated with benzylpenicillin and furosemide (frusemide). Max was also put on a salt and fluid restriction diet to lower the BP and to prevent pulmonary oedema and heart failure. Max made a full recovery 3 weeks later with his BP and renal parameters returning to normal.

Max had nephritic syndrome, characterized by oliguria, mild proteinuria, haema-turia, oedema, and hypertension. Had a kidney biopsy been carried out, it would have shown immune complexes deposited in the glomerular subepithelium. These immune complexes, possibly containing streptococcal antigens can be detected by immuno-fluorescence and would have activated the complement system, which would have attracted neutrophils to the area. The ensuing inflammatory response would have

resulted in glomerular damage resulting in proteinuria, haematuria and hypoalbuminaemia.

What does the positive ASO result indicates? What is the biological function of ASO?
Explain why the C3 levels were low.
Explain the possible mechanism underlying the oedema.
Explain the mechanism underlying the hypertension.

Another major complication of *Streptococcus pyogenes* infection is rheumatic fever,
which was mentioned in Chapter 2.

Trigger box   Nephritic syndrome

Try to work out what the special features mean!
Features: Oliguria, proteinuria, macroscopic haematuria, HTN, mild oedema.
Reduced GFR with elevated urea and creatinine.

Causes:	Special features
Poststreptococcal glomerulonephritis	Lumpy bumpy; ASO; lowC3
IgA nephritis(most common type)	Steroid responsive
Wegener's granulomatosis	cANCA, steroids, cytotoxics
Alport's syndrome	Deafness, boys, hereditary
Goodpasture's syndrome	Haemoptysis, linear anti-GBM deposits

Treatment: Treat HTN, uraemia, fluid overload.
Steroids, immunosuppresive drugs.

John's diabetic kidney

An event that involved John further highlights the importance of maintaining the
integrity of the glomerular basement membrane. Some 15 years after being diagnosed
as a type 2 diabetic, John too had to visit the Renal Unit at Hope Hospital. His disease
was affecting his kidneys.

At the renal unit John was found to have ankle oedema. There was also loss of ankle
pulses, absent ankle jerks and some loss of foot sensation. Urinalysis revealed heavy
proteinuria but no glucose. Subsequent 24 hour urine protein excretion was 6.5 g. An
mid-stream urine sample (MSU) showed no evidence of infection. Serum analysis
revealed hypoalbuminaemia, hypoproteinaemia and hypercholesterolaemia, but normal creatinine, urea and electrolytes. A kidney ultrasound was normal.

What do you think is causing these findings?
What is the mechanism of the hypercholesterolaemia?

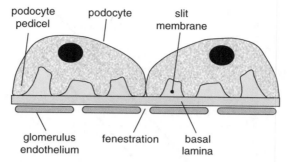

Figure 4.7 Ultrastructure of the glomerular filtration barrier. Adapted from Tortora and Grabowski (2003), Principles of Anatomy and Physiology, 10th edition, John Wiley & Sons

A renal biopsy showed nodular glomerulosclerosis with a thickened GBM, mesangial expansion and Kimmelsteil–Wilson nodules. John was showing evidence of diabetic nephropathy resulting in heavy proteinuria, hypoalbuminaemia, oedema and hypercholesterolaemia: the nephrotic syndrome.

Filtration at the GBM is affected by the size and net charge of filtered substances. In nephrotic syndrome the loss of basement membrane negative charge leads to the loss of plasma albumin. Figure 4.7 shows the glomerular filtration barrier.

Unfortunately things got worse and John returned to the renal unit 3 years later presenting with ankle oedema and nocturia. His BP was 170/97 and his urea and creatinine were raised although the electrolytes were normal. The renal consultant warned against emergent chronic renal failure.

Trigger box Nephrotic syndrome (NS)

Try to work out what the special features mean!

Features: Heavy proteinuria, hypoalbuminemia, hyperlipidaemia, generalized oedema. Dyspnoea, ascites, increased susceptibility to infection, PE, venous thrombosis.

Causes	Special features
Minimal change disease	Most common in children; idiopathic; epithelial foot process fusion
Focal segmented glomerulosclerosis	Idiopathic, IVDA, HIV
Membranous nephropathy	Most common cause of NS in adults; immune complex disease
	HBV, syphilis, malaria; spike & dome
Diabetic nephropathy	Thick GBM, increased mesangial mass, Kimmelsteil–Wilson
Lupus nephritis	Subendothelial immune complexes
Amyloidosis	Multiple myeloma, RA, TB; congo red; apple green birefringence

Treatment: Protein, salt restriction, diuretics, antihyperlipidemics, ACEIs.

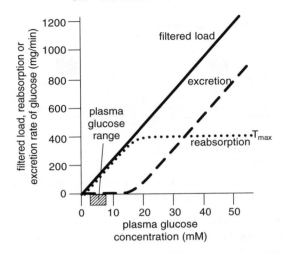

Figure 4.8   Glucose filtration

John did not show any glycosuria during the above visits to the Renal Unit. When he was first diagnosed with type 2 diabetes, however, Dr Smith found glycosuria. This brings us to events occurring after filtration and highlights the process of reabsorption.

John's glycosuria was the result of his rate of glucose filtration rising above the T_{max} (maximum rate of glucose reabsorption) for glucose which normally happens when the plasma glucose is >11 mmol/L. Glucose clearance is shown in Figure 4.8.

Going back to Max...

Let us consider Max's electrolyte findings. Table 4.3 lists the main causes and consequences of electrolyte abnormalities.

Max was hyperkalaemic, hyperphosphataemic and had a metabolic acidosis with respiratory compensation. We can explain these findings by considering what happens to the filtrate once it passes from the Bowman's capsule into the proximal tubule.

Figure 4.9 shows the functions of the key regions of the kidney tubules: the proximal tubule, the loop of Henle, the distal tubule and the collecting ducts. Figure 4.9 also shows the key sites where diuretics work. The properties of key diuretics are shown in Table 4.4.

The proximal tubule is the workhorse of the kidney, and, as seen in Figure 4.9 this is where around 70–80 per cent of the reabsorption of water and Na^+, takes place. Most of the HCO_3^-, glucose and amino acid reabsorption also take place here. Secretion of NH_3, which buffers secreted H^+, also takes place (Fig. 4.10).

The filtrate then passes into the descending loop of Henle. The loop of Henle is responsible for maintaining a concentration gradient of the interstitial fluid, which allows concentration of the urine by the collecting duct. Urine concentration involves the interstitium, the loop and the medullary blood vessels, the vasa recta. The medullary

Table 4.3 Electrolyte abnormalities

Electrolyte disturbance	Common causes	Treatment
Hypernatraemia	*Hypovolaemic* Dehydration due to inadequate fluid intake Diarrhoea/fistulae sweating diabetes insipidus, diabetes mellitus. *Hypervolaemic* Excess mineralocorticoid: Na^+ retention	Rehydration Treat underlying condition
Hyponatraemia: hypervolaemic	Salt and water retention *Urine Na^+ <30 mmol/L* Heart failure Cirrhosis *Urine Na^+ >30 mmol/L* Nephrotic syndrome Renal failure	Diuretics ACEI Angiotensin 2 receptor antagonists Aldosterone antagonists Salt and water restriction
Hyponatraemia: hypovolaemic	Loss of fluid containing Na^+ *Urine Na^+ <30 mmol/L* Diarrhoea/vomiting/fistulae Haemorrhage Sweat, burns, ulcers *Urine Na^+ >30 mmol/L* Renal disease, diuretics Addison's disease	Salt and water replacement Blood Treat underlying condition
Hyponatraemia: euvolaemic	*Urine Na^+ <30 mmol/L* Acute water intoxication *Urine Na^+ >30 mmol/L* Syndrome of inappropriate ADH secretion (SIADH)	Water restriction SIADH: Demeclocycline Treat underlying condition
Hyperkalaemia	*Reduced renal excretion* Renal failure Mineralocorticoid deficiency (e.g. Addison's disease) Drugs – ACEI and potassium sparing diuretics *Intracellular to extracellular K^+ shift* Acidosis Intravascular haemolysis Release from white cells (e.g. leukaemia) and platelets (thrombocytopenia) Familial pseudohyperkalaemia Hyperkalaemic periodic paralysis	Emergency Cardioprotection: slow i.v. calcium Lower plasma K^+: i.v. dextrose-insulin to (ECF K^+ → ICF K^+) Promote K^+ loss: ion exchange resins, dialysis (renal failure) Treat underlying condition

(Continued)

Table 4.3 (*Continued*)

Electrolyte disturbance	Common causes	Treatment

Hypokalaemia	*High urine K^+*
	Diuretics
	Excess mineralocorticoid
	  (e.g. Conn's)
	Renal tubular acidosis
	Diabetic ketosis, metabolic
	  alkalosis
	
	Low urine K^+
	D & V
	Inadequate intake
	
	Extracellular to intracellular K^+ shift
	Alkalosis
	Familial periodic paralysis
		K^+ supplements – oral is preferable to i.v.
		Treat underlying condition

Hypercalcaemia	See Ch. 5	

Hypocalcaemia	*Increased phosphate*
	Chronic renal failure
	* Hypoparathyroidism (includes
	  Mg deficiency)
	Pseudohypoparathyroidism
	Acute rhabdomyolysis
	Tumour hyperphosphataemic lysis
	
	Low/normal phosphate
	Vitamin D deficiency
	Acute pancreatitis
	Pseudovitamin D deficiency
	Hereditary vitamin D resistance
	*All have high PTH except
	hypoparathyroidism
		Emergency
		Ca^{2+} supplements: oral
		  preferable to i.v.
		
		Vitamin D ± calcium
		  supplements treat Underlying
		  condition

Hypomagnesaemia	*Inadequate intake*
	Dietary deficiency
	Malabsorption
	Familial primary hypo-
	  magnesaemia
	
	Renal loss
	Alcoholism
	Diuretics
	Nephrotoxic drugs (cisplatin)
	Familial hypomagnesaemia
	
	Extracellular to intracellular
	  Mg^{2+} shift
	Re-feeding syndrome
		Mg^{2+} supplements
		treat Underlying condition

ACEI, angiotensin converting enzyme inhibitor; D & V, diarrhoea and vomiting; PTH, parathyroid hormone; ADH, antidiuretic hormone.

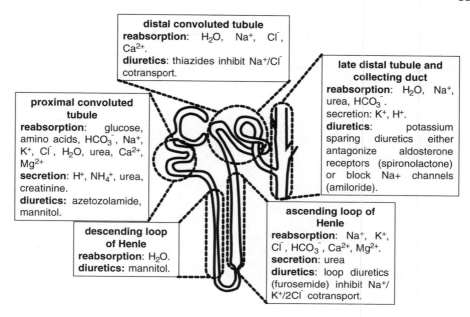

distal convoluted tubule
reabsorption: H_2O, Na^+, Cl^-, Ca^{2+}.
diuretics: thiazides inhibit Na^+/Cl^- cotransport.

late distal tubule and collecting duct
reabsorption: H_2O, Na^+, urea, HCO_3^-.
secretion: K^+, H^+.
diuretics: potassium sparing diuretics either antagonize aldosterone receptors (spironolactone) or block Na+ channels (amiloride).

proximal convoluted tubule
reabsorption: glucose, amino acids, HCO_3^-, Na^+, K^+, Cl^-, H_2O, urea, Ca^{2+}, Mg^{2+}
secretion: H^+, NH_4^+, urea, creatinine.
diuretics: azetozolamide, mannitol.

descending loop of Henle
reabsorption: H_2O.
diuretics: mannitol.

ascending loop of Henle
reabsorption: Na^+, K^+, Cl^-, HCO_3^-, Ca^{2+}, Mg^{2+}.
secretion: urea
diuretics: loop diuretics (furosemide) inhibit $Na^+/K^+/2Cl^-$ cotransport.

Figure 4.9 Tubular functions and diuretics

concentration gradient is maintained by the fact that the descending loop is permeable to water but impermeable to Na^+, K^+ and Cl^-, whereas the ascending limb of the loop is impermeable to water but permeable to Na^+, K^+ and Cl^-.

By means of a diagram explain the countercurrent mechanism that leads to the medullary concentration gradient.

The ascending loop segment also induces reabsorption of Mg^{2+} and Ca^{2+}. Loop diuretics like furosemide (frusemide) act by inhibiting the Na^+, K^+ and Cl^- cotransport system preventing the concentration of urine. These drugs can cause hypocalcaemia and hypokalaemia.

Can you explain why loop diuretics cause hypokalaemia and hypocalcaemia?

Describe the function of the vasa recta

What are juxtamedullary and cortical nephrons? Compare and contrast their structural features and functions.

Let us move on to the distal collecting tubule. This segment, which is impermeable to water, reabsorbs Na^+, Cl^- and Ca^{2+}, the latter regulated by PTH. In the early distal tubule Na^+Cl^- is reabsorbed. This is blocked by thiazide diuretics. These drugs can cause a hypokalaemic metabolic alkalosis, hyponatraemia, and hypercalcaemia.

Table 4.4   Examples of commonly used diuretics

Type	Action	Examples	Indications	Side effects
Thiazides and related diuretics Moderately potent diuretics	Inhibit distal tubule Na^+/Cl^- symporters	Bendroflumethazide, xipamide, indapamide	CHF, HTN	Hypokalaemia, hyponatraemia, hypomagnesaemia, hypercalcaemia, hyperuricaemia, hyperglycaemia, altered plasma lipid levels, alkalosis. Weakness, skin rashes, impotence
Loop diuretics Potent diuretics	Inhibit ascending loop of Henle $Na^+/K^+/2\ Cl^-$ co transporters	Furosemide, bumetanide, torasemide	Renal failure, severe CHF	Hyponatraemia, hypokalaemia, hypocalcemia, hypomagnesaemia, hyperuricaemia and gout, ototoxicity
Potassium-sparing diuretics Weak diuretics	Na^+ channel blocker Aldosterone receptor antagonist Potentiates thiazide or loop diuretics	Amiloride, triamterene (Na^+ channel blocker), spironolactone (aldosterone receptor antagonist)	Digitalis patients, cirrhosis	Hyperkalaemia, hyponatraemia, gynaecomastia
Osmotic diuretics	Increases tubular fluid osmolarity	Mannitol	Cerebral oedema	
Carbonic anhy-drase inhibitors Weak diuretic	$NaHCO_3$ diuresis Reduction of HCO_3^-	Acetazolamide	Used in glaucoma Oedema of pregnancy	

CHF, congestive heart failure; HTN, hypertension.

The collecting tubes reabsorb Na^+ in exchange for K^+ and H^+, which are secreted. This is regulated by aldosterone. Reabsorption of water in the collecting duct is controlled by ADH.

How do thiazides cause hypokalaemic metabolic alkalosis, hyponatraemia, and hypercalcaemia

The collecting tubules are composed of principal cells and intercalated cells. The principal cells are involved in Na^+ reabsorption, K^+ secretion, and water reabsorption; the intercalated cells are involved in K^+ reabsorption and H^+ secretion. K^+ sparing diuretics such as spironolactone and amiloride work in these regions. Spironolactone is

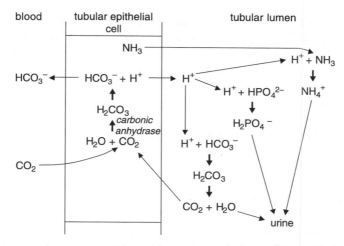

Figure 4.10 Renal regulation of pH. Adapted from McGeown (1999) Physiology, Churchill Livingstone

an aldosterone receptor antagonist in the collecting tubule. Amiloride blocks Na channels in the same region. Therefore they can cause hyperkalaemia.

List the factors that cause secretion of ADH

What is SIADH? Describe the metabolic consequences of SIADH

Trigger box **Diabetes insipidus**

Thirst, polydipsia, polyuria.

Water deprivation test: hyperosmolar with inappropriate dilute urine.

1. *Central*

Failure of pituitary secretion of ADH.

Causes: Tumour, Sheehan syndrome, trauma, infection, autoimmunity.

Investigations: desmopressin acetate (DDVAP) challenge, MRI.

Treatment: intranasal DDVAP.

2. *Nephrogenic*

Kidneys fail to respond to ADH.

Causes: Drugs (e.g. lithium), renal disease.

Treatment: Salt restriction, increase water intake.

Thiazide diuretics.

We can now fully explain Max's laboratory data. When Max had his haemorrhage, the decrease in RBF and GFR reduced the amount of Na arriving at the collecting ducts so reducing the secretion of K^+ and H^+. This caused the hyperkalaemia and metabolic acidosis. The hyperkalaemia gave rise to the ECG changes such as peak T waves.

Max was acidotic and we can now consider the kidneys role in acid-base balance. This involves

- Excretion of H^+

- Generation and recovery of bicarbonate

- Excretion of bicarbonate

- Generation of NH_4^+, $H_2PO_4^-$.

Reabsorption of HCO_3^- and secretion of H^+, plays a major role in the regulation of acid–base balance. Figure 4.10 shows the regulation of pH through renal secretion of H^+ and absorption of HCO_3^-.

H^+ and HCO_3^- are generated in the tubular cells by dissociation of carbonic acid formed by CO_2 and H_2O. This reaction is catalysed by carbonic anhydrase. The H^+ is actively transported to the lumen while the HCO_3^- is ejected into the peritubular capillaries. Filtered HCO_3^- is therefore exchanged for H^+.

Can you explain why Max has decreased bicarbonate levels?
What are the main causes of renal tubular acidosis?

List the main buffer systems found in blood

Describe the kidney's role is producing *new* HCO_3^- via HPO_4^{2-} and NH_3.

Let us look at Max's blood gases. Max's metabolic acidosis led to a compensatory hyperventilation, which resulted in lowering of paCO$_2$ (respiratory compensation). Acidosis and alkalosis was considered in Chapter 2.

The role of the kidney in regulating calcium and phosphate is considered in Chapter 6

Let us return to Max's haemorrhage, which led to acute renal failure. When the paramedics found him his blood pressure was precipitously low. This gives us an opportunity to recall another important kidney function: the regulation of BP. This was considered in Chapter 2.

The decrease in afferent arteriole blood pressure, the reduction in Na^+ in the filtrate and the increase in SNS activity caused by the baroreceptor reflex which has been stimulated by the decrease in blood pressure all lead to stimulation of the juxtaglomerular apparatus (Figure 4.11), which releases renin. Renin cleaves the circulating protein angiotensinogen into angiotensin I which is then cleaved by angiotensin-converting enzyme (ACE) produced in the lung into angiotensin II. Angiotensin II has two functions: a vasoconstriction effect that increases blood pressure and a stimulation of the release of aldosterone. Aldosterone acts on the distal convoluted tubule to

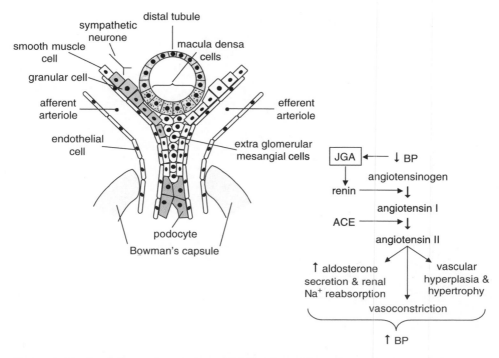

Figure 4.11 Juxtaglomerular apparatus (JGA). Adapted from Tortora and Grabowski (2003), Principles of Anatomy and Physiology, 10th edition, John Wiley & Sons

increase Na^+ and water reabsorption, which also raises blood pressure. These effects however take several hours to develop fully.

Max's dehydration and hypernatremia would have also contributed to the release of ADH.

 What are ACE inhibitors? Describe how they reduce BP?

 Describe the mechanism and significance of tuboglomerular feedback.

 We have described several endocrine functions of the kidney. Two other important hormones that are relevant the kidney are erythropoetin and ANP. Can you describe their functions?

 Describe how serveral neural circuits control the process of micturition.

5

The endocrine system

Learning strategy

The endocrine system consists of several endocrine glands that produce hormones, which have a variety of functions.

A good way to learn the functions of the hormones produced by the endocrine gland is by considering the clinical effects of under- or oversecretion of these key hormones.

As you read the clinical scenarios, it is important to review the normal anatomy, embryology, and physiology of the endocrine glands. In addition to understanding the pathophysiological basis of the disease processes, study of the endocrine system also affords a good opportunity to review the key metabolic pathways involved in carbohydrate and lipid metabolism. Also reviewing the mechanisms of action of the key anti-thyroid and anti-diabetic drugs will help reinforce the metabolic principles underlying the functions of the key hormones involved.

Try to answer the questions and try to complete the Learning tasks.

Mary is slowing down ...

Mary was feeling poorly. For months she had been feeling tired. The weather didn't help; her problems were worse in the winter when she constantly felt cold. 'I am aching all over' she complained to John who was struggling with his own problems 'and my voice has changed'. 'Well you're getting on a bit, Dear' John remarked casually, 'and I like your husky voice'. 'I'm only 50' Mary retorted.

Integrated Medical Sciences   by Shantha Perera, Stephen Anderson, Ho Leung and Rousseau Gama
© 2007 John Wiley & Sons, Ltd   ISBN: 978470016589 (HB) 978470016596 (PB)

Debbie, who was listening to all this made things worse by remarking that she was also gaining weight. Mary groaned. She was feeling rather depressed of late and Debbie's comment didn't help. Mary made a mental note to see Dr Smith the next morning.

Dr Smith observed her as she began going over her many concerns. She looked tired. He noticed that her eyes were puffy and her arms and hands were dry and pale. Her voice was hoarse and her hair appeared coarse and dry.

Her BP was 138/89, pulse 65, regular. Her respiratory examination was unremarkable, although her respiratory rate was 23.

Dr Smith already had an inkling of her problem. He palpated her thyroid: it was enlarged and somewhat hard. He ordered some tests which arrived a week later.

The results of Mary's initial investigations are shown in Table 5.1.

'Looks like you have an underactive thyroid, Mary' Dr Smith told her when she

Table 5.1 Mary's results

Free thyroxine (FT4)	4 pmol/L (12.0–22.0)
Free tri-iodothyronine (FT3)	1.8 pmol/L (3.95–6.8)
Thyroid-stimulating hormone (TSH)	72.3 mU/L (0.25–4.25)
Thyroid peroxidase antibody titres	Strongly positive

attended the surgery the following week. I am going to refer you to Dr Hobbit. He is an endocrinologist. He may suggest you to have a needle biopsy".

Mary's problem sets the stage to begin our exploration of the endocrine system. Figure 5.1 shows the location of the major endocrine glands and indicates the hormones produced.

In this chapter we will discuss the pituitary, the thyroid, the adrenals and the pancreas. The parathyroid glands will be covered in Chapter 6. The reproductive glands will be covered in Chapter 7.

Let us look at the origins of the endocrine glands. The pituitary is the 'master gland' and has two distinct lobes: anterior and posterior (Figure 5.2). The anterior lobe develops from the ectodermal Rathke's pouch, which forms the adenohypophysis, the intermediate lobe and the pars intermedia. The diencephalon forms the posterior lobe.

The thyroid gland is derived from the epithelium in the floor of the tongue and descends to its final position. The pancreatic islets of Langerhans develop in the third month within the pancreatic tissue. Insulin secretion starts around the fifth month.

The adrenal cortex develops from mesoderm, whereas the medulla develops from ectoderm. After birth the fetal cortex undergoes regression and only its outermost layer remains. Neural crest cells invade the adrenal cortex and give rise to the medulla. These are the chromaffin cells that produce catecholamines.

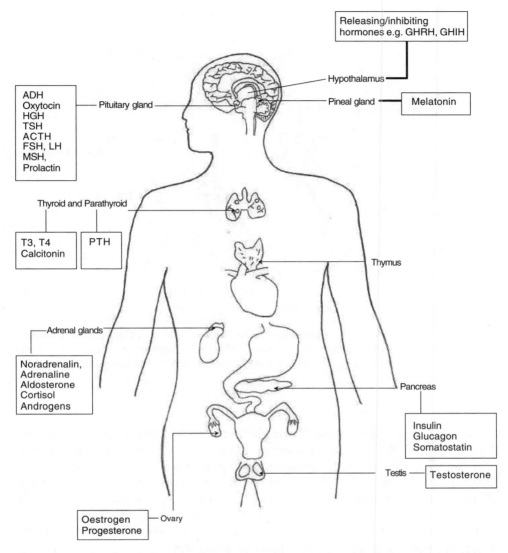

Figure 5.1 Location of the endocrine glands and hormones produced. Note that the kidney produces calcitonin and erythropoetin. The GI tract produces gastrin, secretin, cholecystokinin and GIP

Craniopharyngioma is a tumour arising from remnants of the Rathke's pouch. What are its features and what kind of symptoms does it produce?
Neuroblastomas can be found in the abdomen. Can you explain this observation?

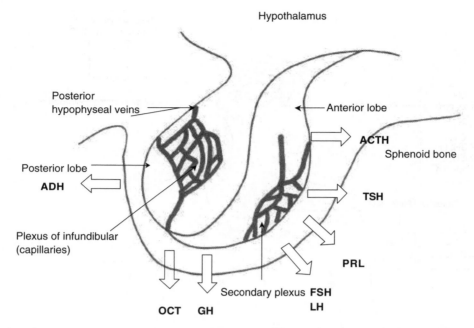

Figure 5.2 The anatomy and hormones of the pituitary gland. ACTH, adrenocorticotro-pic hormone; TSH, thyroid-stimulating hormone; FSH, follicle-stimulating hormone; LH, lu-teinizing hormone; PRL, prolactin; GH, growth hormone; ADH, antidiuretic hormone; OCT, oxytocin

Let us start our exploration of the glands by briefly considering the pituitary. Figure 5.1 also indicates the release hormones produced by the hypothalamus that stimulate secretion of the pituitary hormones, which are also indicated in the figure. In this chapter we will discuss the pituitary hormones: growth hormone (GH), thyroid stimulating hormone (TSH) and adrenocorticotropic hormone (ACTH), the latter two when we look at the thyroid and adrenals. Follicle-stimulating hormone (FSH) luteinizing hormone (LH), prolactin and oxytocin will be discussed in Chapter 8. ADH (and diabetes insipidus) was discussed in Chapter 4.

We will start with human growth hormone (hGH). hGH secretion is regulated by two hypothalamic hormones: growth hormone releasing hormone (GHRH), which stimulates secretion, and growth hormone inhibiting hormone (GHIH), which inhi-bits secretion. hGH is a major anabolic hormone and stimulates the growth of bone and soft tissue. Growth is modulated by insulin-like growth factors (somatomedins) released by the liver upon response to hGH. hGH is crucial for growth during child-hood and adolescence. It is also an insulin antagonsist and may increase blood glucose levels.

A usually benign pituitary growth hormone secreting adenoma raises hGH levels causing acromegaly.

> ### *Trigger Box* Acromegaly
>
> Benign pituitary adenoma secreting GH.
>
> **Excess GH effects:** Coarse facial features, prognatism, large tongue, soft tissue enlargement, large feet, 'spade-like' hands, carpal tunnel syndrome, hypertension, goitre, glucose intolerance.
>
> **Tumour effects: Intrasellar** – hypopituitarism.
>
> **Extrasellar extension** – headaches, visual field defects, cranial nerve palsies, rhinorrhoea. Increased mortality from cancer and cardiovascular disease.
>
> **Investigations:** Failure of GH suppression during oral glucose tolerance test (OGTT). 25% have diabetes on OGTT
>
> MRI – pituitary tumour.
>
> **Treatment:** Pituitary surgery, radiotherapy, somatostatin and its analogues, dopamine agonists (bromocriptine), pegvisomant (GH receptor antagonist).
>
> NB Children with excess hGH have *gigantism*.

? *What are the main clinical consequences of panhypopituitarism?*

Let us now consider the thyroid gland in more depth. The formation of the thyroid hormones is shown in Figure 5.3. Iodide ions pumped into the colloid combines

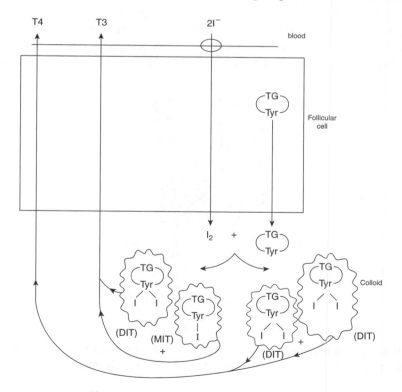

Figure 5.3 Formation of thyroid hormones

Table 5.2   Thyroid hormone functions

Linear growth and maturation of bone (stimulates GH secretion)
Development of central nervous system
Increased BMR
Increased glycogenolysis, gluconeogenesis, lipolysis
Increased CO, HR, SV, contractility, respiration rate (RR), O_2 consumption

with tyrosine (attached to thyroglobulin) forming monoiodotyrosine (MIT) and diiodotyrosine (DIT). T3 and T4 are formed from the combination of MIT and DIT. The functions of the thyroid hormones are shown in Table 5.2.

Mary's lab data illustrates the important principle of feedback, which is a characteristic of the regulation of endocrine function. For example, in the case of the thyroid, the hypothalamus produces thyrotropin-releasing hormone (TRH), which causes the anterior pituitary to release TSH that in turn causes the release of the thyroid hormones T3 and T4. The increased level of thyroid hormones negatively feedbacks on TSH and TRH causing their levels to decline. Figure 5.4 shows the feedback loops.

What are the main arteries supplying the thyroid?
What is the possible mechanism causing Mary's goitre?

Mary ended up in Hope Hospital Outpatients. Sitting in reception, waiting to be called into Dr Hobbit's office she wished she could have had a small drink to steady her nerves; she was worried about the needle biopsy result. Then she spotted one of her old school friends, Paula. It was years since she had seen her – they weren't really close friends at

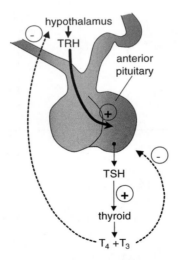

Figure 5.4   Thyroid hormone feedback loops. Adapted from Tortora and Grabowski (2003), Principles of Anatomy and Physiology, 10th edition, John Wiley & Sons

school but she had bumped into her a few times shopping in town. Mary moved over to her and said hello. Paula was pleased to see Mary and soon they were chatting away.

While talking to Paula Mary noticed that her school friend had changed a lot. First of all her eyes appeared to be sticking out. She looked a little sweaty and her hands were trembling a bit. She also had a bulge in her neck. Mary was surprised when Paula mentioned that she too had thyroid problems and that she was a regular at Dr Hobbit's clinic. 'I've got an overactive thyroid' she remarked. 'Dr Hobbit put me on carbimazole but that made my thyroid gland underactive and I had to be put on thyroxine. Still, if the carbimazole didn't work I would probably have had surgery to remove my thyroid gland.'

> *Why do some patients get hoarse after thyroid surgery? Which nerve has the surgeon got to be careful about?*
> *What is the mechanisms of action of carbimazole?*
> *What is thyroid storm? How is it treated?*

Their conversation was interrupted by the buzzer, which called Mary in to see Dr Hobbit. Dr Hobbit read the needle biopsy report – it indicated fibrosis and a lymphocyte infiltration – and informed Mary of the diagnosis: Hashimoto's thyroiditis. He explained the autoimmune basis of Mary's thyroid gland problem and prescribed thyroxine.

Table 5.3 lists some key organ specific and organ non-specific autoimmune diseases. Complete Table 5.3 by indicating the autoantigens.

Table 5.3 Autoimmune diseases

Disease	Autoantigen
Organ-specific diseases	
Addison's disease	
Autoimmune haemolytic anaemia	
Goodpasture's syndrome	
Hashimoto's thyroiditis	
Graves' disease	
Type 1 diabetes mellitus	
Idiopathic thrombocytopenic purpura	
Myasthenia gravis	
Multiple sclerosis	
Pernicious anaemia	
Non-organ specific diseases	
Ankylosing spondylitis	
Rheumatoid arthritis	
Systemic lupus erythematosus	
Sjögren's syndrome	
Scleroderma	

> Define central and peripheral tolerance. Describe putative mechanisms that might lead to autoimmunity.

Hashimoto's thyroiditis is an example of a primary hypothyroidism where the gland itself is compromised owing to autoimmune destruction. Congenital thyroid hormone deficiencies and iodine deficiency can also cause a primary hypothyroidism. In cretinism there is inadequate development of the brain due to thyroid hormone deficiency in the first months of life.

In secondary hypothyroidism, the levels of TSH are reduced due to deficient secretion from the pituitary as occurs in hypopituitarism. This then causes deficient T3 and T4 production. The thyroid gland usually atrophies because of the low TSH levels.

Hyperthyroidism can also be due to primary, or very rarely secondary, causes. In Paula's case stimulatory autoantibodies cause the excessive production of T3 and T4 reducing TSH levels. This is Graves' disease. The stimulation of the gland can cause goitres.

Trigger box   **Thyroid diseases**

1. *Hypothyroidism* (myxoedema)
   Features: Lethargy, mild weight gain, constipation, cold intolerance, dry skin, puffy face, hair loss, deep, hoarse voice, bradycardia, slow relaxation of reflexes, psychosis, dementia, myxoedema coma, myxodema madness.
   Findings: High TSH, low T4, autoantibodies.
   Treatment: Thyroxine for life.

   Causes
   A. *Hashimoto's thyroiditis*; autoimmune; thyroid microsomal antibodies, atrophy, goitre.
   F > M; late middle age.
   Hypothyroid or euthyroid. Initially may be hyperthyroid.

   B. *Iatrogenic*
   Following radioiodine or thyroid surgery.

   C. *Iodine deficiency*
   Mountain regions.
   Goitre, euthyroid or hypothyroid.

   D. *Congenital*

2. *Hyperthyroidism*
   Features: Increased appetite but weight loss, irritability, hyperkinesis, sweating, palpitations, tachycardia (atrial fibrillation), tremor, diarrhoea.
   Thyroid storm: Hyperpyrexia, tachycardia, delirium, coma, death.
   Treatment: Carbimazole, propanolol, dexamethasone.
   Findings: High FT4 and FT3 and suppressed TSH.

Causes

A. *Graves' disease*

IgG to TSH receptor. Elevated thyroid microsomal & thyroglobulin autoantibodies. Predominantly young women.

Also diffuse goitre, thyroid eye disease (exophthalmos, lid retraction, chemosis), pretibial myxoedema, onycholysis and other autoimmune diseases.

Thyroid radionucleotide scan: Diffuse uptake.

Treatment: Carbimazole, radioactive iodine, surgery.

Propanolol for initial control of symptoms.

B. *Toxic adenoma, toxic multinodular goitre*

Thyroid nodule(s) may be palpable.

Older age-group.

Thyroid radionucleotide scan: localised uptake ('hot nodule').

Treatment: Radioactive iodine, surgery, carbimazole.

Zoe's moon face...

Unlike Debbie, Zoe never remarked on Mary's weight problems. This was because she was also having the same problem: she was getting fat. Over the last 6 months she had put on 10 kg and was being teased at school. Just the other day Debbie had remarked that her face was becoming rounder.

Zoe's brittle asthma was getting worse in spite using maximum doses of three different inhalers most of the time. She was 14 years old now and had been suffering from asthma since age 6. She had had to visit the emergency doctors for acute asthma frequently and even had to be admitted to hospital on three occasions. She was treated with many courses of prednisolone, a synthetic corticosteroid. The prednisolone was then tapered off when she returned home. But no sooner had this happened than she got another asthma attack, which meant going back on the steroids and eventually ended up taking prednisolone more or less continuously. Zoe finally confided her concerns to Mary who took her to see Dr Smith.

Dr Smith noticed the weight gain and the general change in Zoe's demeanour. She looked moodier than usual, and was extremely reticent. She had acne and some facial hirsutism. Dr Smith also noticed some cervical fat padding and red striae on her abdomen, breasts and inner thighs. Her BP was 143/94, pulse 87/min regular. The rest of the physical exam was normal. Reviewing her growth charts, Dr Smith noted that her growth velocity had dropped and her height was in the 3rd percentile. Her weight however had increased. He ordered an endocrinology screen.

These revealed that Zoe's ACTH was very low as was her endogenous cortisol. The rest of the endocrinology screen was normal.

Can you explain Zoe's lab data?

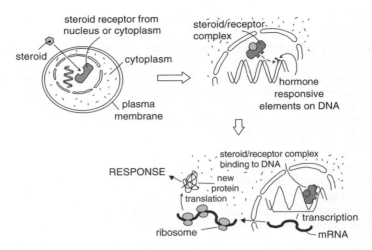

Figure 5.5 Steroid mechanism of action. Adapted from Rang, Dale, Ritter and Moore, (2003) Pharmacology, 5th edition, Churchill Livingstone

Dr Smith realized that her long-term asthma and oral prednisolone treatment had to be managed more carefully and referred her to a paediatrician at Hope hospital.

This scenario leads us to consider another important steroid hormone, cortisol, and the gland that produces it: the adrenal. Figure 5.5 shows the mechanism of action of steroids.

The structure of the adrenal gland is shown in Figure 5.6 Note the two regions and the hormones produced by them. In this chapter we will focus mainly on cortisol and the mineralocorticoid aldosterone which we also considered in Chapter 4. The androgens will be described in Chapter 7.

In order to understand Zoe's results we need to consider the hypothalamus–pituitary –adrenal (HPA) axis, which is shown in Figure 5.7 Her over-use of exogenous cortisol (prednisolone) was suppressing her HPA axis, which resulted in a suppression of her ACTH, which in turn decreased her natural cortisol levels. Table 5.4 shows the metabolic functions of cortisol.

Cortisol has a permissive effect on catecholamines. Glucocorticoids are important in promoting glycogenolysis driven by catecholamines (epinephrine and norepinephrine). Also the cardiovascular responses mediated by catecholamines require glucocorticoids.

The anti-inflammatory role of glucocorticoids is exemplified by Zoe's requirements to control her asthma, which, as described in Chapter 1, is an inflammatory disease. Additionally corticosteroids also inhibit B- and T-cell responses and have been used to suppress specific immune responses in transplantation.

Zoe was becoming Cushingoid due to the effects of excessive administered cortisol. Cushing's syndrome could be iatrogenic (as in Zoe's case), due to a pituitary adenoma secreting ACTH, ectopic ACTH secretion from a non-pituitary tumour, or due to an adrenal tumour secreting cortisol, all of which can cause elevated levels of glucocorticoids.

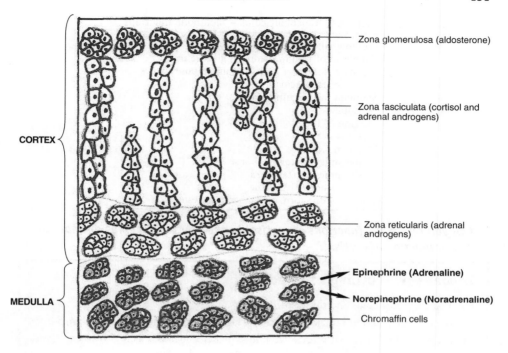

Zona glomerulosa (aldosterone)

Zona fasciculata (cortisol and adrenal androgens)

CORTEX

Zona reticularis (adrenal androgens)

Epinephrine (Adrenaline)

Norepinephrine (Noradrenaline)

MEDULLA

Chromaffin cells

Figure 5.6 The histology of the adrenal gland

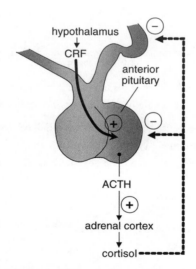

Figure 5.7 The HPA axis. Adapted from Tortora and Grabowski (2003), Principles of Anatomy and Physiology, 10th edition, John Wiley & Sons

Table 5.4   Glucocorticoids – metabolic functions

Promote gluconeogenesis
Inhibition of insulin mediated glucose uptake
Facilitate storage of fat in certain adipose tissues
Release of fatty acids
Maintain muscle function
Wakefulness
Increase GFR
Fetal maturation
Maintain CO
Inhibit inflammatory response
Inhibit immune responses
Decrease connective tissue
Decrease bone formation; increases resorption

? *Can you relate the functions of cortisol to the physical findings of under and overproduction of cortisol?*

Trigger box   Cushing's syndrome

Elevated glucocorticoids and mineralocorticoids.
Features: Central obesity, buffalo hump, moon face (plethoric), thin bruisable skin, purple striae, acne, HTN, proximal muscle weakness, diabetes mellitus, depression, psychosis, amenorrhoea/oligomenorrhoea and decreased libido and erectile failure in men.
Diagnosis: Loss of cortisol diurnal rhythm.
Increased 24 h urine free cortisol.
Failure of cortisol to suppress during 1 mg overnight dexamethasone suppression test.
Causes

1. *High ACTH*

a. Cushing's disease: Pituitary microadenoma secreting ACTH causing bilateral adrenal hyperplasia.
Exaggerated cortisol and ACTH responses to corticotropin release factor (CRF).
Partial suppression of cortisol during high dose dexamethasone suppression.

b. Ectopic ACTH due to tumours such as carcinoid, small cell lung cancer.
No cortisol and ACTH responses to CRF.
No suppression of cortisol during high dose dexamethasone suppression.

2. *Suppressed ACTH*

a. Adrenal tumours.
No suppression of cortisol during high dose dexamethasone suppression.

b. Iatrogenic Cushing's (exogenous glucocorticoids).
Treatment: Surgery.
Metapyrone, ketoconazole (cortisol inhibitors).
Iatrogenic: Reduce steroids to minimal effective dose for minimum possible time.

Describe the dexamethasone suppression test and its uses in the diagnosis of Cushing's disease

Let us look at mineralocorticoid excess. Hyperaldosteronism can be primary or secondary. Primary hyperaldosteronism (Conn's syndrome) is most often due to a unilateral adrenal adenoma (65 per cent) but may also be due to bilateral adrenocortical hyperplasia (30 per cent). The Trigger box below shows the key features of Conn's syndrome. It might be useful to review the renin–angiotensin–aldosterone axis which is shown in Chapter 2.

Trigger box   Conn's syndrome (primary hyperaldosteronism)

Clinical features: Resistant hypertension, headache, polyuria, muscle weakness.

Findings: hypokalaemia with alkalosis, inappropriate kaliuresis.

Diagnosis: Elevated plasma aldosterone cannot be suppressed by fludrocortisone or saline infusion.

Low (often suppressed) plasma renin activity. Therefore high aldosterone:renin ratio. CT/MRI adrenals.

Main causes: Adrenal adenoma (65%), bilateral adrenal hyperplasia (30%).

Treatment: Adrenalectomy for adenoma, Spironolactone for bilateral hyperplasia.

What are the causes of secondary hyperaldosteronism?

Note: Secondary hyperaldosteronism: *high* renin and *high* aldosterone.

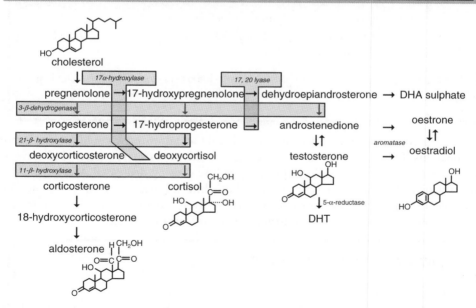

Figure 5.8 Steroid metabolism pathways. Adapted from Ganong (1991) Review of Medical Physiology, 15th edition, Appleton & Lange

Let us briefly consider adrenal hyperplasia. In a congenital type of adrenal hyperplasia there is an increase in adrenal androgens and cortisol deficiency. Figure 5.8 shows the steroid pathways in the adrenal gland and indicates the consequences of key enzyme deficiencies. The most common is a 21-hydroxylase deficiency. Other causes of cortisol deficiency include 11 hydroxylase and 17 hydroxylase deficiencies. The deficiency of cortisol stimulates ACTH synthesis, which in turn leads to the overproduction of other steroids notably adrenal androgens.

Trigger box   Congenital adrenal hyperplasia

Common features: Cortisol deficiency.
hyperpigmentation (high ACTH), bilateral adrenal hyperplasia and overproduction of other steroids (eg androgens) prior to block.
Increased androgens can cause ambiguous genitalia in female infants; virilization (late), macrogenitosomia, precocious puberty.
Lab findings: Cortisol deficiency. High levels of cortisol precursors (17 hydroxyproges-terone) and androgens.

21-hydroxylase deficiency (AR)
Most common (95%)
Features as above and salt wasting and hypotension in 75% patients (due to mineralocorticoid deficiency.
Lab findings: High levels of cortisol precursors, androgens.

11β-hydroxylase deficiency and 17α-hydroxylase deficiency
As above and hypertension and hypokalaemia due to increased mineralocorticoid precusors (deoxycorticosterone).

Treatment: Hydrocortisone for cortisol deficiency which also reduces ACTH and hence androgens
Surgery.

If Zoe's corticosteroid treatment was suddenly withdrawn she could go into acute adrenal insufficiency. Adrenal insufficiency could be primary (adrenal disease – Addison's disease) or secondary (pituitary failure causing decreased ACTH produc-tion). Cortisol production is reduced in both but aldosterone production may be reduced in Addison's disease whereas it is relatively unaffected in pituitary failure because the renin–angiotensin–aldosterone axis remains unaffected.

Trigger box   Adrenal insufficiency

Addison's disease
Destruction of adrenal cortex by autoantibodies, tumours, tuberculosis, intra-adrenal haemorrhage.

In autoimmune Addison's disease, the major autoantigen is the adrenal enzyme, 21-hydroxylase, and rarely 17α-hydroxylase. Associated with other autoimmune diseases.

Features: Lethargy, depression, nausea, vomiting, weight loss, hyperpigmentation, vitiligo, loss of body hair, postural hypotension.

Lab findings: Hyponatraemia, hyperkalaemia, uraemia, hypoglycaemia, eosinophilia, neutrophilia,

Addisonian crisis: hypovolaemic shock, abdominal pain.

Diagnosis: Synthetic ACTH (Synacthen) test – inadequate rise in cortisol.

Treatment: Lifelong steroid treatment (hydrocortisone, fludrocortisone). Increase dose during stress.

Can you explain why patients have hyponatraemia and hyperkalaemia?

The Synacthen test is used to diagnose primary and secondary adrenocortical failure. A test dose of Synacthen (synthetic ACTH analogue) will not increase cortisol levels in primary and secondary insufficiency.

Max's terrible headache ...

The above discussion illustrates the functioning of the adrenal cortex. We can now turn to the adrenal medulla by considering what happened to Max one night.

One evening the family was awakened by the telephone. It was Debbie, who was staying with Max at the time. Max was back in hospital. Apparently he had visited the emergency GP with a terrible headache earlier that evening. Max was also nauseous and had vomited several times that evening. He had been covered in sweat and his heart was racing. He had had similar but less severe episodes in the past few weeks.

The physician had noted a greatly raised BP of 200/105, and had immediately sent Max to the ED.

What could account for Max's symptoms?

A CT scan revealed a mass in the left adrenal gland. The most common primary tumour of the adrenal gland is called a phaeochromocytoma. This is derived from chromaffin cells in the adrenal medulla and secretes adrenaline (epinephrine) and noradrenaline (norepinephrine). Overproduction of these hormones leads to the observed symptoms. Max's phaeochromocytoma was confirmed by three consecutive 24-h urine tests that measured metanephrines, urinary free catecholamines, and their metabolites (e.g. vanillylmandelic acid, VMA).

Max was also found to be hyperglycaemic Can you explain the mechanism?
What are the main effects of adrenaline? Why is adrenaline called the fight-or-flight hormone?

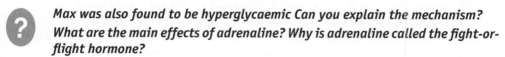
Describe how catecholamines are formed and how they are broken down by catechol-o-methyl transferase and monoaminooxidase. What are monoamine oxidase inhibitors?

Trigger box   **Phaeochromocytoma**

SNS tumour (0.1% of HTN).

Causes

90% Adrenal	10% Extra-adrenal
90% Benign	10% Malignant
90% Unilateral	10% Bilateral
90% Sporadic	10% Inherited

Some associated with multiple endocrine neoplasia (MEN).

Clinical features: Hypertension (persistent, paroxysmal, orthostatic).

Triad: Headache, sweating and palpitations.

Hyperglycaemia.

Diagnosis: Increased 24 h urine free catecholamines (adrenaline, noradrenaline, dopamine) and their metabolites.

Increased plasma metanephrines.

CT/MRI, metaiodobenzylguanidine scan (MIBG).

Treatment: Alpha (phenoxybenzamine), beta (propanolol) blockade before surgery (why is this necessary?).

Which conditions constitute type 1 and type 11 multiple endocrine neoplasia?

Little John can't stop drinking ...

Six months later things were improving at Sunnybrook Cottage. Mary's thyroid symptoms had abated and Zoe's asthma attacks were getting much less frequent. Both mother and daughter were also losing some weight. Max's surgery had gone well and he was back to his usual self.

Then, when the family was just about to breathe a collective sigh of relief ... Little John became ill.

Two days after his 10th birthday Mary found Little John lethargic. and running a temperature. He had a bad cough and was coughing up yellow–green sputum. In fact he had been feeling tired and had been oversleeping for the past 4 weeks. Little John was also drinking constantly was always complaining of thirst. He had also mentioned that his vision was blurry. Mary took him to see Dr Smith.

Dr Smith examined Little John. He was underweight for his age and looked drowsy. He looked pale and sweaty and his skin looked dry. His BP was 115/65 but his HR was 96 bpm. He was breathing deeply and rapidly at 38 per min. Auscultation revealed crackles in his left lung base. As he moved closer Dr Smith noted that his breath smelled sweet.

What is most likely causing his lung crackles?
What is causing his sweet-smelling breath?

Table 5.5 Little John's results

PH	7.20 (7.36–7.44)
H^+	63 nmol/L (36–44 nmol/L)
PaO_2	14.0 kPa (9–13 kPa)
$PaCO_2$	2.0 kPa (4–6 kPa)
HCO_3^-	10 mmol/L (22–25 mmol/L)
Glucose	32 mmol/L (<11.1 mmol/L)
Na^+	150 mmol/L (135–145 mmol/L)
K^+	6.1 mmol/L (3.5–5.0 mmol/L)
Creatinine	0.12 mmol/L (0.06–0.13)

Realizing that he was dealing with a medical emergency, Dr Smith arranged Little John to be taken to the hospital.

Little John was diagnosed with suffering from a chest infection, which had triggered a diabetic ketoacidosis. Blood was drawn for analysis and he was rehydrated vigorously with intravenous fluids and commenced on insulin infusion and intravenous flucloxacillin.

The blood results are shown in Table 5.5.

What are the consequences of raised serum potassium?
Why was Little John later treated with KCl?

Little John was started on insulin injections in hospital. The paediatrician, explained to John and Mary that Little John was suffering from type 1 diabetes and hence had a deficiency of insulin due to the actions of anti-pancreatic islet cell antibodies, which were destroying his pancreatic islets. The diabetic nurse specialist spent a lot of time on the ward with the family explaining to them the importance of following the dietary advice and taught them capillary blood glucose monitoring for when he went home.

Can you explain why Little John has almost no insulin but John senior has near normal levels in spite of them both suffering from diabetes?

Little John is suffering from type 1 diabetes; his dad John on the other hand is a type 2 diabetic. Both conditions involve insulin, the key anabolic hormone secreted by the pancreatic islets of Langerhans which also secretes glucagon and somatostatin.

Insulin and glucagon are primarily involved in the regulation of blood glucose. Somatostatin inhibits the release of insulin. However, these hormones significantly affect most metabolic pathways involving carbohydrate and lipid metabolism (see Chapter 3).

 List the other key functions of somatostatin.

Tables 5.6 to 5.8 show the main features and metabolic functions of insulin, glucagon and the counter-regulatory hormones adrenaline and cortisol. These are called counter-regulatory hormones because they oppose the effects of insulin.

Table 5.6   Insulin: features and key metabolic functions

Proinsulin is cleaved to release insulin and C-peptide.
Insulin release stimulated mainly by portal blood glucose levels and some amino acids.
Insulin peaks after 30–45 min after eating and returns to baseline within 2 to 4 h.
No effect on glucose uptake by brain, RBCs and hepatocytes.
Promotes cellular glucose uptake through glucose transporters (GLUTs).
GLUT 1 found in brain and erythrocytes; GLUT 2 found in liver and pancreatic β1 cells.
GLUT 3 found in brain and placenta, GLUT 4 found in skeletal muscle, cardiac muscle and
    adipose tissue.
Promotes glycogenesis and inhibits glycogenolysis.
Stimulates glycolysis and pyruvate oxidation.
Inhibits gluconeogenesis.
Stimulates pentose-phosphate shunt (PPP).
Promotes lipogenesis.
Inhibits lipolysis and ketogenesis.
Increases protein synthesis and cell growth.
Increases cholesterol synthesis.

Table 5.7   Glucagon: features and key metabolic functions

Peptide.
Secretion stimulated by low plasma glucose and high amino acid and adrenaline (epinephrine)
levels. Glucagon is therefore decreased in response to a carbohydrate meal and elevated during
fasting.
Stimulates gluconeogenesis.
Suppresses glycogenesis.
Increases glycogenolysis.
Stimulates lipolysis and ketogenesis.
Suppresses lipogenesis.
Inhibits cholesterol synthesis.

Table 5.8   Adrenaline and cortisol: relevant metabolic functions

Adrenaline is released during acute stress.
Cortisol is released during chronic stress and fasting.

Adrenaline
Decreases glycogenesis.
Promotes glycogenolysis in muscle and liver.
Stimulates fatty acid release from adipose tissue.

Cortisol
Stimulates gluconeogenesis.
Stimulates fatty acid release from adipose tissue.
Stimulates amino acid mobilization from muscle protein.

What is the relevance of C peptide measurement in clinical practice?

Little John suffers from type 1 diabetes mellitus whereas John has type 2 diabetes mellitus. The trigger box below shows the key features of this important disease and table 5.9 shows the interpretation of the oral glucose tolerance test.

Trigger box Diabetes	
Type 1	Type 2
Usually peaks at puberty (<30 years)	Usually after 40 years
Lean, HLA DR3/DR4, 40% concordance	Overweight, Asians/blacks, 50% concordance
Pathogenesis: autoimmune destruction of β cells (e.g. antibodies vs GAD), insulitis, insulin resistance, complete insulin deficiency, associated with autoimmnue diseases.	Pathogenesis: relative insulin deficiency & resistance.
2–4 week history of polyuria, polydipsia, lethargy, weight loss.	Symptoms over months, vulvitis, balanitis (candida), visual problems, lethargy
Diabetic ketoacidosis (DKA).	Hyperosmolar hyperglycaemic non-ketotic coma (HONK).

We can now understand the biochemical basis of Little John's signs and symptoms. Little John's DKA was due to increased fatty acid production due to enhanced lipolysis. The lack of insulin promoted lipolysis resulting in ketogenesis. Ketone metabolism is shown in Figure 5.9.

The unopposed stimulation of the counterregulatory hormones adrenaline and cortisol also contributed to the observed ketogenesis.

Once you have reviewed the metabolic effects of these hormones you should be able to work out the answers to the following questions.

Why was Little John losing weight?

What do you think are the possible mechanisms underlying Little John's polyuria and polydipsia?

Table 5.9 The 75G oral glucose tolerance test

	Plasma Venous Glucose (mmol/L)		
	Fasting		120 min
Normal	<6.1	&	<7.8
Impaired fasting Glycaemia	≥6.1–<7.0	&	<7.8
Impaired GTT	<7.0	&	≥7.8–<11.1
Diabetes Mellitus	≥7.0	&/or	≥11.1

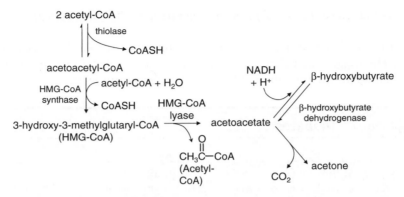

Figure 5.9 Ketone metabolism. Adapted from Stryer (1988), Biochemistry, 3rd edition, Freeman

Why was he hyperkalaemic and acidotic?

Why was he sweaty? And why was his HR increased?

Why was his BP low?

One day, several years later Little John forgot to eat after taking his regular insulin jab. After playing football he collapsed. The paramedics gave him an IM injection of glucagon. What was the rationale of this treatment?

John's losing control...

A few weeks later John visited Dr Smith. John was dismayed about Little John's type 1 diabetes. Despite reassurances from Dr Smith, he was convinced that he was somehow responsible for his son's condition. While at the surgery, Dr Smith checked him out. In fact his routine visit was long overdue.

History revealed some visual problems, intermittent claudication and patchy loss of sensation in several toes.

Dr Smith enquired about his glycaemic control. Although John hadn't been keeping a regular check he felt that his glucose levels were under control. A urine test confirmed this but Dr Smith found proteinuria. Dr Smith also noted ankle oedema and loss of ankle pulses. There was some sensory loss in several toes and an ulcer was spotted on his left shin. His BP was 160/92. Fundoscopy revealed hard exudates and dot-blot haemorrhages. Dr Smith ordered an HbA1c test.

What is the basis of this test? What information will it provide Dr Smith?

John's type 2 diabetes is due to insulin resistance. List the possible mechanisms of insulin resistance?

Table 5.10   Diabetic complications

Complication	Physical findings
Microvascular	
Retinopathy	dot-blot, cotton wool spots, ,
Neuropathy	Peripheral: sensory, loss of vibration sense, absent ankle jerks
	Autonomic dysfunction
Nephropathy	Proteinuria
Macrovascular	
Cardiovascular disease	Angina, MI
Cerebrovascular disease	Stroke, TIA
Peripheral vascular disease	Intermittent claudication (absent pedal pulses)

John was showing signs of chronic diabetic complications a possible consequence of his poor glycaemic control. Table 5.10 shows the main complications and their associated physical findings.

Table 5.11   Diabetes treatment strategies

1. *Biguanides* Reduce hepatic glucose production, primarily gluconeogenesis (e.g. metformin), Metformin does not promote weight gain and has beneficial effects on several cardiovascular risk factors. Side effects: GI disturbance, lactic acidosis
2. *Sulphonylureas* stimulate insulin secretion (older and cheaper sulfonylureas, e.g. glipizide, glimepiride. Newer and more expensive rapid-acting secretagogues such as meglitinides e.g. repaglinide and nateglinide) Side effect: hypoglycaemia
3. *Alpha-glucosidase inhibitors (AGIs)* delay digestion and absorption of intestinal carbohydrate (e.g. acarbose and miglitol) side effect: GI disturbance
4. *Thiazolidinediones, TZD* increase target cell response to insulin (e.g. rosiglitazone and pioglitazone). Side effect: hepatotoxicity

Insulin is required for:
1. Survival in type 1 diabetes mellitus
2. Glycaemic control in type 2 diabetes if life-style and oral anti-diabetes medication has not achieved glycaemic targets
3. Metabolic decompensation such as incipient or actual diabetic ketoacidosis, or non-ketotic hyperosmolar hyperglycaemia
4. In some circumstances, for example pregnancy or severe hepatic or renal impairment
5. In certain co-morbidities such as following myocardial infarction or during acute intercurrent illness

Types of insulin
Almost all are synthetic (recombinant) human insulin
1. *Soluble insulins* start working in 30–60 min; last 4–6 h, use in DKA
2. *Rapid acting insulin* (insulin lispro/aspart) acts in 15 min lasts for 2–4 h. use as pre-meal bolus
3. *Prolonged acting insulins* (glargine, lente); can be intermediate (12–24 h) or long acting (>24 h)

How does enzymatic and non-enzymatic glycosylations of key proteins contribute to diabetic complications?

Dr Smith reviewed John's medication and strongly advised him on the importance of maintaining good glycaemic control. Table 5.11 shows the main anti-diabetic drugs.

'But I am well' John retorted.' Not like poor Little John'. Dr Smith replied that although he was unlikely to develop a ketoacidoisis or a hypoglycaemic coma, he could develop HONK.

'What on earth is HONK?' John asked.

Dr Smith explained that extreme high levels of glucose can cause cause a non-ketotic hyperosmolar coma (HONK).

What is the mechanism underlying HONK?

6

The musculoskeletal system

Learning strategy

In this chapter we will consider the essential, 'must know' features of the muscu-loskeletal system. A brachial plexus injury will introduce you to the upper extremity and a lower limb compartment syndrome to the lower extremity. The main muscu-loskeletal structures of the head, neck and abdomen will be covered by considering scenarios involving clinical examination of these regions. This will then lead us to muscle types, ultrastructure and the physiology of contraction.

A Colles fracture with underlying osteoporosis will lead us to consider bone ultra-structure, embryology and the physiology of calcium and phosphate metabolism.

We will also consider the pathophysiological mechanisms of several key musculo-skeletal/rheumatological diseases which will, in addition to highlighting the key pathological principles, further reinforce basic anatomy, physiology and biochem-istry of the musculoskeletal structures involved.

We will review the key drugs involved in the treatment of common rheumatic diseases.

We will also use the opportunity to review the key blood vessels and nerves supplying the musculature.

Try to answer the questions and try to complete the Learning Tasks.

Max and the motorcycle...

Max was out trying out his brother's motorcycle. He wasn't an experienced rider, and in spite of advice to the contrary, decided to test the considerable acceleration powers of the

Integrated Medical Sciences   by Shantha Perera, Stephen Anderson, Ho Leung and Rousseau Gama
© 2007 John Wiley & Sons, Ltd   ISBN: 978470016589 (HB) 978470016596 (PB)

machine. On a bend Max hit a wet spot on the road and lost control. Soon he was hurtling through the air, landing heavily, hitting the tip of his left shoulder on the tarmac.

Fortunately a car was trailing Max, and the driver witnessed the accident. He stopped his car and ran to the scene. Max was lying on the road a few feet from his mangled bike. He was conscious. The man called the ambulance.

The paramedics found Max lying on his back. He was groaning and in pain. Max complained that he was unable to move his left arm and that his chest, left foot and right knee were hurting. The paramedics placed a brace around his neck to immobilize his cervical spine and fixed a traction splint around his left leg. He was then placed on a stretcher and taken into the ambulance where he was given oxygen by mask, and morphine. His respiration rate was 38 breaths per minute and his BP was 150/95. He was tachycardic (102).

On arrival at the ED Max was examined by the duty consultant and his team. Max complained about the unremitting pain.

The doctors examined his chest; percussion, breath sounds and vocal resonance were normal and there was equal lung expansion, which made a pneumothorax unlikely. A chest X-ray however revealed a cracked left fourth rib.

Max's left arm was hanging at the side with the elbow extended and the forearm pronated. Abduction of the arm at the shoulder appeared to be totally lost, as was external rotation and elbow flexion suggesting that the roots of the fifth and sixth cervical nerves had been torn away from the spinal cord. There were no obvious skull injuries.

Max's left ankle was swollen. Pulses on left ankle and foot were weak, but sensation was normal. The right knee examination was normal, as was the abdominal examination.

The doctors began monitoring his urine output. Blood tests revealed that Max's Hb concentration; haematocrit, WCC and platelet counts were all within the normal range. Blood biochemistry was also normal. All X-rays apart from the chest PA were also normal.

Max's arm was placed in an abduction splint with a movable joint at the elbow.

This scenario introduces us to the musculoskeletal system. We will begin by considering the gross skeletal anatomy and the major muscle groups.

The secondary survey carried out by the doctors of the ED involved a head-to-toe check for abnormalities such as fractures, dislocations, contusions and deformities.

First, they checked Max's skull for injuries. A good way to learn the main bones of the skull is to consider the bones that make up the orbit. As shown in Figure 6.1 several skull bones contribute to form the bony orbit. Other must-know facts about skull anatomy include the key landmarks of the anterior, middle and posterior fossae (e.g. the main foramina), the anatomy of the temporomandibular joint and the sinuses. We are generally oblivious to the sinuses until they become inflamed.

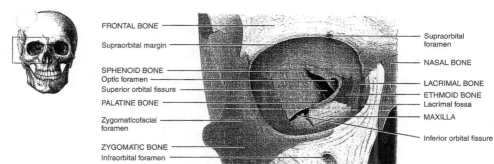

Anterior view showing the bones of the right orbit

Figure 6.1 Orbital bones. Adapted from Tortora and Grabowski (2003), Principles of Anatomy and Physiology, 10th Edition, John Wiley and Sons Inc. New York

---

Trigger box   Sinusitis

Maxillary sinus mostly.

Pathogens:

Acute: Viruses, *Streptococcus pneumoniae, Haemophilus influenzae, Moraxella catarrhalis.*
Chronic: Anaerobes, *Mucor* in diabetes mellitus.

Features: Obstruction of drainage, undrained pus, tenderness, fever, facial pain (can radiate to upper teeth), headache, nasal congestion.

Risk factors: Barotrauma, allergic rhinitis, asthma, smoking.

Investigations: Transillumination, radiology.

Treatment:

Acute: May settle without treatment. Painkillers, decongestants, amoxicillin/trimetho-prim-sulfamethoxazole (TMP-SMZ), doxycycline, erythromycin.
Chronic: Amoxicillin, surgical drainage.

Complications: Osteomyelitis, meningitis, abscess, orbital cellulitis, cavernous sinus thrombosis.

It is important to understand the functioning of the major muscles of mastication, the muscles of facial expression, and the muscles that move the eyeball and eyelids (Figure 6.2).

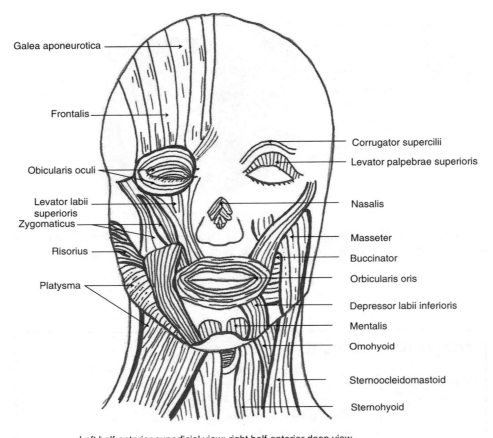

Left half-anterior superficial view; right half-anterior deep view

Figure 6.2 Facial muscles

Which muscles are involved in:

Opening the eyelids
Closing them gently
Closing them tightly
Smiling
Which cranial nerves innervate these muscles?

Complete Table 6.1.

The paramedics were careful to stabilize Max's neck to protect the cervical spine in case there was a cervical spine injury. It is important to know the anatomy of the spinal column particularly the structure of the atlas, axis and the cervical vertebrae and the location of the main neck muscles.

Table 6.1 Muscles of mastication. Complete the table

Action	Muscle(s) involved	Nerve supply To muscle	Arterial supply To muscle
Opening the jaw			
Closing the jaw			

 Compare and contrast the anatomical features of a typical cervical, thoracic and lumbar vertebra.

 If, following the accident Max couldn't turn his head to the right and also had a drooping left shoulder, which nerve is damaged? Which muscles are innervated by this nerve?
Which muscles are used in flexion and extension of the neck?

Max sustained injuries to the upper roots of the brachial plexus (C5 and C6). These resulted in a condition known as Erb–Duchenne palsy (Waiter's tip), which affects the suprascapular nerve and musculocutaneous nerve, and causes paralysis of the rotator cuff muscles, biceps, brachialis, coracobrachialis, and deltoid. The condition is also seen in newborns with shoulder dystocia.

 What constitutes the rotator cuff?

As a result of this injury, the upper limb was hanging limply, medially rotated by the unopposed action of the pectoralis major muscle, and pronated due to a loss of biceps action. The limb is therefore constantly adducted and medially rotated. However, the limb cannot be abducted because both supraspinatus, which initiates abduction, and deltoid, which carries out complete abduction, have been denervated.

The brachial plexus is shown in Figure 6.3, which also indicates the main types of injuries that result from lesions. Study of the brachial plexus injuries should allow revision of the main muscles, bones, nerves and blood vessels of the shoulder region.

 What is Klumpke's palsy?

When testing motor power in the upper extremity elbow flexion and extension, shoulder adduction/abduction, hand extension and flexion, are formally tested by asking the patient to resist the movements elicited by the examiner.

Table 6.2 shows the prime mover muscles involved in the key movements of the upper extremity. The innervation of the muscles is also indicated.

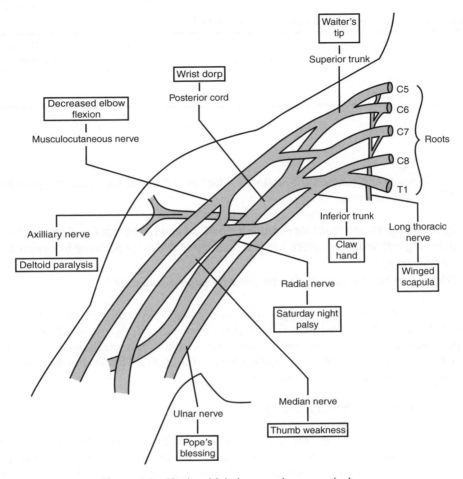

Figure 6.3   The brachial plexus and common lesions

Which muscles and nerves are involved in thumb opposition?

Standard upper extremity reflexes tested in a neuromuscular examination include the biceps, triceps, and brachioradialis reflexes. Which nerves are stimulated when the reflexes are tested? Which nerve roots? Which muscles carry out the movements? Construct a table which can be used for rapid revision.

Find out the main features of the following: shoulder joint; elbow joint; wrist joint.

Table 6.2 The upper extremity

Action	Main muscle(s)	Nerve supply
Arm abduction	Deltoid	Axillary
Arm adduction	Pectoralis major	Pectoral
	Latissimus dorsi	Thoracodorsal
Upper arm extension	Latissimus dorsi	Thoracodorsal
Upper arm flexion	Pectoralis major	Pectoral
Lower arm flexion	Biceps brachii	Musculocutaneous
	Brachialis	Musculocutaneous
	Brachoradialis	Radial
Lower arm extension	Triceps brachii	Radial
Pronation	Pronator teres	Median
	Pronator quadratus	Median
Supination	Biceps brachii	Musculoskeletal
	Supinator	Radial
Wrist flexion	Flexor carpi radialis	Median
	Palmaris longus	Median
	Flexor carpi ulnaris	Ulnar
Wrist extention	Extensor carpii radialis	Radial
	Extensor carpii ulnaris	Radial
Finger extenstion	Extensor digitorum	Radial
Finger flexion	Flexor digitorum superficialis	Median
	Flexor pollicis longus	
	Flexor digitorum profundus	Median
		Ulnar/median

Can you identify these muscles in a diagram? Test yourself.
Following Max's upper extremity injury there would most likely be diminished skin sensation over which part of the upper limb?

In examining sensation the dermatomes are tested methodically. The dermatomes are shown in Figure 6.4.

If Max's humerus was fractured midshaft which nerve and which artery are most likely to be damaged?
If Max had had an anterior dislocation of his shoulder which nerve is most likely to have been damaged?

Max had a fracture in his fourth left rib. It is important to understand the general layout of the ribs, the thoracic vertebrae, the sternum, the scapula and the clavicle.

Which rib is opposite the angle of Louis?

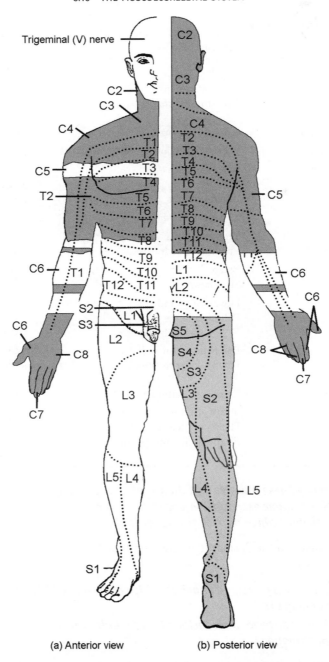

(a) Anterior view   (b) Posterior view

Figure 6.4 The dermatomes. Adapted from Tortora and Grabowski (2003), *Principles of Anatomy and Physiology*, 10th Edition, John Wiley and Sons Inc. New York

During another altercation some years earlier Max suffered from a pneu-mothorax and the doctors had to introduce a chest tube between his second and third rib. Why is it important to pierce the skin above but not below a rib when carrying out this procedure?

Let us now consider the main muscles forming the anterior abdominal wall.

While carrying out the abdominal examination one of the doctors scratched Max's abdomen then pressed and released quickly. 'No guarding or rebound tenderness' she said.

What is guarding and rebound tenderness?
Which abdominal muscles would contract if there were guarding/rebound?
What does it indicate?

The Sickalotts went to visit Max. While waiting in reception Zoe developed another one of her asthma attacks. She began breathing rapidly and had to sit hunched up with her elbows on a table. She was using her accessory muscles. This scene, which we have already come across in Chapter 1, will allow us to review some of the major muscles of the thorax.

Can you name the accessory muscles Zoe is using?
Which muscles are involved in normal and forced inspiration? Which ones are involved in forced and normal expiration?

More problems for Max

As the day progressed Max developed increasing left leg pain. He called out to a passing doctor who examined his leg. The leg was swollen and tender over the posterior, anterior and lateral aspects. Pedal pulses were weak but present.

Which two arteries are commonly palpated when foot pulses are examined?

Motor power was reduced in these leg muscles. There was also decreased sensation in the deep and superficial peroneal nerve distributions. Active ankle plantar flexion and inversion were present but weak due to pain. Capillary filling of the skin of the leg and foot was normal.

When testing motor power in the lower extremity hip flexion and extension, knee flexion and extension, ankle extension and flexion, thigh adduction and abduction are formally tested by asking the patient to resist the movements elicited by the examiner.

Table 6.3 shows the prime mover muscles involved in the key movements of the lower extremity. The innervation of the muscles are also indicated.

Can you identify these muscles in a diagram? Test yourself!!

Table 6.3   The lower extremity

Action	Main muscles(s)	Nerve supply
Thigh extension	Gluteus maximus	Inferior gluteal
	Hamstrings	Sciatic
Thigh flexor	Iliopsoas	Femoral
	Sartorius (rotation also)	Femoral
Knee extension	Quadriceps	Femoral
Knee flexion	Hamstrings	Sciatic
Foot dorsiflexor	Tibialis anterior	Deep peroneal
Foot plantiflexor	Gastrocnemius	Tibial
	Soleus	Tibial
Foot evertor	Peronius tertius	Deep peroneal
	Peronius longus/brevis	Superficial peroneal
Foot invertor	Tibialis posterior	Tibial
	Tibialis anterior	Deep peroneal
Thigh adductor	Adductor longus, magnus and brevis	Obturator & sciatic
	Pectinius (rotation also)	Femoral
	Gracilis(rotation also)	Obturator
Thigh abductor	Glutes medius	Superior gluteal

Standard lower extremity reflexes tested in a neuromuscular examination include the knee and the ankle jerk. Which nerves are stimulated when the reflexes are tested? Which nerve roots? Which muscles carry out the movements? Construct a table which can be used for rapid revision.

Max was suffering from compartment syndrome and since all passive motions of the ankle and toes were exquisitely painful several compartments were likely to be involved. The doctor mentioned the need for a four-compartment fasciotomy.

What is the layout of the musculature of the leg? What are the 'compartments'? Which muscles, were likely to be involved in Max's compartment syndrome?

Max was complaining of knee pain. One of the doctors examined the knee joint again. 'Your ACLs and PCLs are fine' she said.

What are the PCLs and the ACLs?
How is the drawer test carried out?

Draw a sketch figure showing the anatomy of the knee joint.

What is the femoral triangle? Which muscle forms the walls of this triangle?

The open book...

While Max was lying in the ED, a man who had fallen from a tree was brought in to an adjacent cubicle. After examining him and reviewing his X-rays, one of doctors mentioned that he had an open book pelvic fracture.

Describe the main features of the pelvis. Which features allow distinction between a male and a female pelvis?

Compare and contrast direct and indirect hernia.

What are the main anti-gravity muscles that enable us to climb stairs and rise from a sitting position?
Which muscles form the pelvic floor?

John's done his back in!

One day, not long after Max's accident Mary came home from shopping to find John lying on the sofa. He appeared to be in agony. 'I've done me back in' he groaned. 'Probably will have to go off sick again.' 'Well you'll have to go and see Dr Smith, won't you?' Mary said rather unsympathetically.

Low back pain is a very common problem. Table 6.4 lists the main causes of low back pain.

Table 6.4   Low back pain

Mechanical causes	Trauma
	Postural back pain (sway back)
	Muscular and ligamentous pain
	Spondylosis
	Facet joint syndrome
	Disc prolapse
	Spinal and root canal stenosis
	Spondylolisthesis
	Fibromyalgia
Inflammatory causes	Infection
	Ankylosing spondylitis/sacroiliitis
Metabolic causes	Osteoporotic crush fracture of the spine
	Osteomalacia
	Paget's disease
Neoplastic causes	Metastases
	Multiple myeloma
	Primary bone tumours

NB, Main cause is idiopathic!!

Trigger box   **Spinal stenosis**

Middle age–elderly

Pathology: Stenosis of lumbar or C spine: compresses nerve roots.

Most common cause: degenerative joint disease.

Features: Neck pain, back pain radiating to buttocks and legs.

Pseudo/neurogenic claudication

Investigations: X-ray, CT, MRI.

Treatment: NSAIDs, epidural steroid injections.
          Surgical laminectomy.

Dr Smith asked John to bend forward, backwards and rotate his trunk from side to side. He was examining his range of movements.

?   *Which muscles are being used by John to extend, flex and rotate his spine?*

Dr Smith then tested John's ability to passively raise his legs while lying down.

Dr Smith asked John the following questions.

'Where is the pain? (John indicated his lower back – midway between his anterior–superior iliac spines).

Does the pain run down your leg?

John said no. (Had he answered in the affirmative it could have indicated sciatica.)

?   *What is sciatica? What is the most likely cause of sciatica?*

'Are your water-works OK? (John nodded yes). Any numbness around the back passage? (John answered no). These last questions were checking for cauda equina syndrome.

Trigger box   **Cauda equina syndrome**

Pathology: Lesion distal to L1; damages lumbar and sacral nerve roots of cauda equina.

Commonest cause; prolapsed disc.

Features: Flaccid paralysis, sacral numbness (saddle parasthesia), urinary retention, impotence.

?   *John's back pain was most likely due to a sprain of his paraspinous muscles. Where are these located and what are their functions?*

One of the rare causes of low back pain is ankylosing spondylosis. In this condition there is fusion of joints of the spine leading to a condition called bamboo spine. These patients would have limited mobility of the trunk. In late disease, flexion of trunk would be greatly impaired.

Trigger box   Ankylosing spondylosis

Pathology: Chronic inflammation of spine/pelvis, sacroiliitis, may also cause asymmetric peripheral arthritis and enthesitis.
Male, 20s 30s family history.
HLA B27.
Features: Back pain, limitation of spinal movement and reduction in chest expansion. Bamboo spine, Pain worse with inactivity/morning, anterior uveitis, aortitis, 3rd degree heart block.
Investigations: Schober test, X rays.
Treatment: Anti-inflammatories (NSAIDs, corticosteroids, sulfasalazine) and anti-resorptives (bisphosphonates), exercise.

Ninety per cent of cases of ankylosing spondylitis are associated with HLA B27 (major histocompatibility complex 1).What does this association tell you about the putative pathophysiological mechanism of this disease?

We can now consider the main types of muscle. The structure of smooth, striated and cardiac muscle is shown in Figure 6.5. Compare and contrast the main structural and physiological features of these three types of muscle.

Skeletal muscles can be further subdivided into slow twitch (type I fibres) and fast twitch (type II fibres). Slow twitch fibres are found mainly in postural muscles where slow sustained contractions take place. These fibres use oxidative metabolism to generate the ATP required for contraction. They therefore contain lots of mitochondria and are fatigue resistant. They are red due to presence of myoglobin.

What is the function of myoglobin?

The fast twitch fibres can be further subdivided into IIA and IIb subtypes. Type IIA or fast oxidative fibres also use oxidative metabolism. Examples are calf muscles. They are

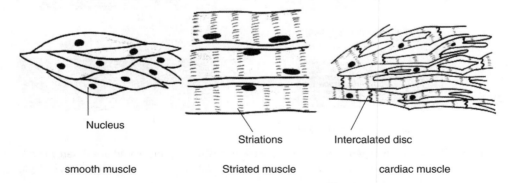

Nucleus

Striations   Intercalated disc

smooth muscle   Striated muscle   cardiac muscle

Figure 6.5   Smooth, striated and cardiac muscle

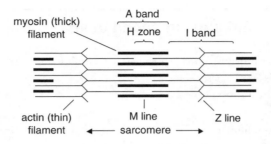

Figure 6.6   Ultrastructure of a myofibril

moderately fatigue resistant. Type IIB or fast glycolytic fibres are white and rely on anaerobic metabolism. They are fatigue fast. Examples are extraocular muscles.

Let us now look at muscle ultrastructure. Skeletal muscle is composed of muscle cells or fibres. A muscle fibre is composed of a series of parallel myofibrils. The ultrastructure of a myofibril is shown in Figure 6.6 The thick and thin myofibrils slide across one another during contraction. This sliding filament theory of muscle contraction is shown in Figure 6.7. Figure 6.8 shows the contraction cycle that causes the filaments to slide.

Describe the mechanisms involved in twitch and tetanic contraction.

Describe isotonic and isometric contractions.

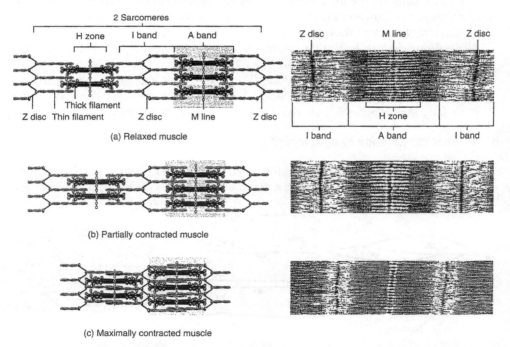

Figure 6.7   Sliding filament-mechanism of muscle contraction in two adjacent sarcomeres. Adapted from Tortora and Grabowski (2003), Principles of Anatomy and Physiology, 10th Edition, John Wiley and Sons Inc. New York

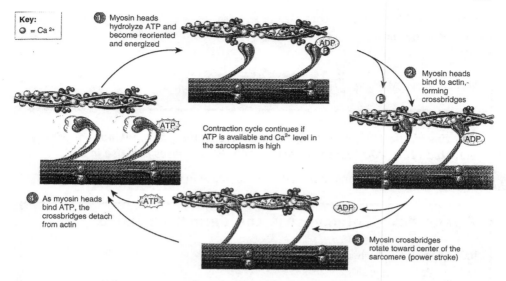

Figure 6.8   The contraction cycle (full credit line). Adapted from Tortora and Grabowski (2003), Principles of Anatomy and Physiology, 10th Edition, John Wiley and Sons Inc. New York

The boy in the wheelchair

Max was relieved. 'Boy! I am glad I didn't break my neck' he told Debbie.' I would have ended up like poor Toby.' He was referring to Toby Brown, one of his old school friends, who was in a wheelchair. Toby however did not end up in a wheelchair because of a spinal injury. He suffered from Duchenne muscular dystrophy, which is an X-linked disease where there is a lack of dystrophin, a protein that connects the cytoskeleton of muscle to the extracellular matrix. Lack of dystrophin leads to severe muscle weakness.

Trigger box   Duchenne muscular dystrophy (DMD)

X-linked recessive disorder.

Absence of dystrophin on immunochemical staining.

1/3 of cases are spontaneous mutants.

1:3000 male infants.

Clinically obvious by fourth year, severely disabled by 10 and often death by 20.

Initial proximal limb weakness with pseudohypertrophy of the calves.

Difficulty in running.

Gowers' sign: patient uses his hands to climb up his leg when he tries to rise to an erect position from the floor.

The myocardium is affected.

Creatine kinase (CK) is grossly elevated (100–200× normal).

Muscle biopsy.

EMG shows a myopathic pattern.

Supportive treatment.

Wheelchair bound by 13.

What is Becker MD?

Creatine kinase (CK), previously known as creatinine phosphokinase, is grossly elevated (100–200 times normal) in DMD. What causes this rise in CK?

List other conditions that lead to an increase in CK levels.

Trigger box   **Polymyositis and dermatomyositis**

Inflammation and necrosis of skeletal muscle.

1/3 have dermatomyositis.

Polymyositis commoner in adults, dermatomyositis relatively common in children.

Symmetrical proximal (shoulder/pelvic girdle) muscle weakness, dysphagia.

Weakness, wasting, pain and tenderness of muscles.

Associated with underlying malignancy, myocarditis, arrhythmias and interstitial pulmonary fibrosis.

Dermatomyositis: Heliotrope rash, Grotton's papules (pathognomonic), Raynaud's syndrome.

Increased serum CK and aldolase.

EMG shows fibrillations.

Investigations: Anti-Jo-1, MRI.

Treatment: Prednisolone, immunosuppressives.

Prognosis better in adults.

Monitor malignancy.

Irene's dinner fork...

Two months later Irene fractured her wrist. She was out shopping with Mary when she tripped and fell onto her outstretched hand.

At the ED an X-ray confirmed a radial fracture. The doctor noticed a bump on the dorsum of the wrist produced by the radius being displaced posteriorly. 'You have a Colles' fracture' the doctor said to Irene.' We call it a dinner fork deformity'. Irene was marginally impressed by this last comment.

He plastered her arm, took some blood for tests and suggested she have her bone density measured.

Table 6.5 Biochemical features in common disorders of calcium and bone metabolism

Disorder	Calcium	Phosphate	ALP	PTH	Other features
Osteoporosis	N	N	N	N/H	–
Primary hyperparathyroidism	H	L	N/H	H	–
Humoral hypercalcaemia of malignancy	H	L	N	L	High parathyroid hormone related peptide (PTHrP)
Bone metastases	H	N	H	L	–
Multiple myeloma	H	N	N	L	Paraprotein in blood & urine
Primary hypoparathyroidism	L	H	N/H	L	–
Pseudohypoparathyroidism	L	H	N	H	–
Pseudopseudo- hypoparathyroidism	N	N	N	N	–
Renal osteodystrophy	L	H	N/H	H	High serum creatinine
Osteomalacia	L/N	L/N	H	H	Low serum vitamin D
Paget's disease	N	N	N	H	–

L, low; N, normal; H, high.

Where is the anatomical snuffbox?

Irene's laboratory tests indicated that her serum calcium and phosphate levels were within the normal range. Her alkaline phosphatase levels were, however, elevated; the doctor suggested that this could be due to the fracture. Table 6.5 shows biochemical features in common disorders of calcium and bone metabolism.

Let us now consider bone structure and formation. The structure of a long bone is shown in Figure 6.9. Cortical or compact bone, which represents 80 per cent of the mass, is found in the shafts of the appendicular skeleton. Trabecular or spongy bone is mainly found in the axial skeleton (vertebrae, ribs, skull, and pelvis).

Bone is mesodermal in origin. In most bones mesenchymal cells differentiate into cartilage cells, the chondrocytes, which secrete a matrix and so produce a cartilaginous model of bone. At a *primary ossification centre* the chondrocytes cells disintegrate and trabecular bone is then deposited on the cartilaginous remnants. This is called endo-chondral ossification. In long bones *secondary centres of ossification* appear at the epiphyses. Growth in the epiphyses is called interstitial growth and is responsible for increasing the length of the bone. Increase in bone diameter is achieved by new bone

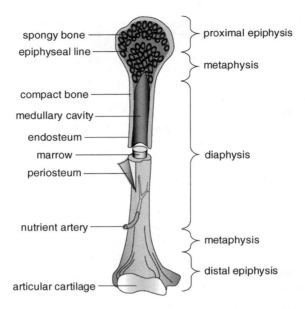

Figure 6.9   Structure of a long bone. Adapted from Tortora and Grabowski(2003), *Principles of Anatomy and Physiology*, 10th edition, John Wiley and Sons

being laid down by the osteogenic layer of the periosteum. In other bones (e.g. membrane bones found in the skull) mesenchymal cells become bone directly (intra-membraneous ossification).

What differences would you see in a normal X-ray of the arm taken from John (51) and little John (10)?

Describe the processes involved in the healing of Max's broken rib?

What do you understand by the terms: healing by primary and secondary intention?

Bone is formed on the outer surface of cortical bone and resorption occurs in its inner surface. During growth, formation exceeds resorption and growth occurs in the epiphyseal growth plates. These plates close off at the end of *adolescence*.

Total bone mass peaks between 20 and 30 years. After 50 years resorption exceeds formation so bone mass decreases.

The main cells of bone are the osteoblasts, osteocytes and osteoclasts. Bone is formed by osteobasts, which make and secrete type 1 collagen, which creates the osteon. Table 6.6 shows details about these cells.

Where do you find Type 1, 2, 3 and 4 cartilage?

Excessive collagen and fibrin deposition throughout the body is the hallmark of scleroderma.

Table 6.6 Functions of cells in bone tissue

Cell type	Derivation	Location	Function
Osteogenic cell	Mesenchyme	Inner periosteum, endosteum, bone canals containing blood vessels	Unspecialized cells that undergo division to produce osteoblasts.
Osteoblast	Osteogenic cells	Within bone matrix	Synthesis and secretion of collagen fibres and the formation of the organic matrix of bone. Begins to initiate calcification.
Osteocyte	Osteoblast	Entrapped within bone matrix it created as an osteoblast	Send out processes into canaliculi to connect with other osteocytes. Exchanges nutrients and wastes with blood.
Osteoclast	Fusion of up to 50 monocytes	Concentrated around the endosteum	Release of acids to dissolve calcium phosphate deposits and lysosomal enzymes to digest the organic matrix, so reabsorbing bone.

Trigger box **Scleroderma**

Multisystemic disease.

Commonly seen as the CREST (Calcinosis, Raynaud's, Oesophageal dismobility, sclerodactyly, telangiectasia) syndrome.

Females 30–50.

Severe disease features: pulmonary fibrosis, cor pulmonale, acute renal failure (ARF), HTN.

Investigations: Anticentromere antibodies (CREST). Anti Scl-70 (systemic).

Treatment: Steroids, ACEIs, calcium blockers (Raynaud's).

Calcium phosphate and hydroxyapatite is deposited within the osteon. Sixty per cent of bone weight is due to calcium hydroxyapatite. The mineralization of bone requires normal plasma concentrations of Ca and PO_4. Vitamin D is involved in the regulation of

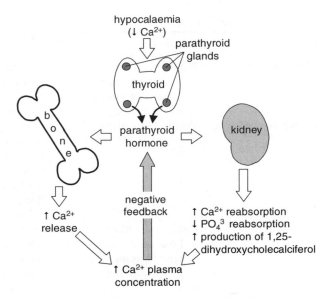

Figure 6.10   Role of the kidney in calcium homeostasis. Adapted from Tortora and Grabowski (2003), *Principles of Anatomy and Physiology*, 10th edition, John Wiley and Sons

Ca and PO_4 metabolism, as shown in Figures 6.10 and 6.11. Vitamin D deficiency causes rickets in children and osteomalacia in adults. The most important hormone involved in Ca and PO_4 metabolism is parathyroid hormone (PTH).

PTH is produced by chief cells of the parathyroid glands, which develop from branchial pouches between 5 and 14 weeks of fetal life.

PTH increases plasma calcium levels by increasing bone resorption (stimulating osteoclasts and osteoblasts); increasing distal kidney calcium reabsorption; and indirectly increasing gut calcium absorption by increasing 1,25 $(OH)_2$ vitamin D production by stimulating kidney 1-α-hydroxylase activity. PTH decreases serum PO_4 by decreasing proximal tubular reabsorption of PO_4.

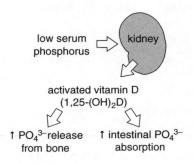

Figure 6.11   Phosphate homeostasis. Adapted from Tortora and Grabowski(2003), *Principles of Anatomy and Physiology*, 10th edition, John Wiley and Sons

Trigger box Rickets and osteomalacia

Pathology: Poor mineralization of osteoid due to vitamin D deficiency.

Causes of vitamin D deficiency: Privation, lack of sunlight, dietary deficiency, malabsorption, chronic renal disease (loss of vitamin D1 hydroxylase), anticonvulsants, inborn errors of metabolism.

Findings: Low serum vitamin D, hypocalcaemia, hypophosphataemia, high parathyroid hormone, increased alkaline phosphatase, Looser's zones (pseudofractures).

Treatment: Oral vitamin D.

Features of rickets: Craniotabes (thin deformed skull at birth), widened epiphyses at the wrists, beading at the costochondral junctions ('rickety rosary'), groove in the rib cage (Harrison sulcus).

In older children, lower limb deformities and myopathy.

Features of adult osteomalacia: Bone or muscle pain and tenderness.

Proximal myopathy – 'Waddling gait'.

Fractures are rare and usually asymptomatic.

Tetany, fits and prolonged QT interval on ECG due to hypocalcaemia.

Brittle bone boy with blue eyes...

One of Little John's classmates, Kevin also had a bone disease, which caused his bones to be very brittle. He was always having fractures, which occurred with minimal trauma and was at one time thought to be a victim of child abuse. Kevin also had noticeable blue sclerae. He was, in fact, suffering from osteogenesis imperfecta.

Trigger box Osteogenesis imperfecta

Phenotypically and genetically heterogeneous.

Most common pathology: type 1 collagen synthesis defect (AD).

Pathology: Abnormal collagen synthesis.

Features: Multiple fractures, brittle bones, blue sclerae.

How is this condition managed?

? *What is the role of calcitonin in calcium metabolism?*

Trigger box Hyperparathyroidism

Hypercalcaemia due to excess PTH.

Adenoma, hyperplasia, carcinoma can cause primary hyperparathyroidism.

Renal failure, vitamin D deficiency causes secondary hyperparathyroidism.

Findings: Severe hypercalcaemia – malaise, depression, bone pain, abdominal pain, nausea, constipation, polyuria, nocturia, renal calculi, renal failure CNS effects, cardiac arrest.
Treatment: Surgery.
Acute; bisphosphonate infusion.
Other causes of hypercalcaemia: malignancy, sarcoidosis, excess vitamin D, milk-alkali syndrome, mutiple myeloma, breast cancer, thiazides, Addison's disease.

The results of Irene's bone density measurement indicated that she had postmenopausal osteoporosis. She was advised to stop smoking and exercise more and was started on calcium and vitamin D supplements and bisphophonates.

Trigger Box: **Osteoporosis**

Decreased bone mass (low bone density); disruption of bony microarchitecture

Features

Increased fractures: Low-trauma fractures e.g. vertebral crush fracture, Colles', fractures of the neck of the femur.

Risk factors

Reduced physical activity, smoking, advancing age, ethnicity (Caucasians and Asians), poor nutritional status, hypogonadism (including menopause), excessive alcohol intake, family history, low body weight, medication (e.g. corticosteroids), systemic disease.

Types

Type 1 or postmenopausal

Due to hypogonadism (i.e. oestrogen or testosterone deficiency).

Oestrogen deficiency causes bone to become more sensitive to the effects of parathyroid hormone (PTH).

Results in accelerated bone loss due to increased osteoclast activity.

Osteoclast (via action of TNF-α and interleukins 1 and 6) production by mononuclear cells may be increased in the presence of gonadal deficiency.

Type 2 or senile osteoporosis

Decreased formation of bone and decreased renal production of 1,25(OH)$_2$ D3. Loss of cortical and trabecular bone and increased risk for fractures.

Type 3 osteoporosis

Secondary to medications, e.g. glucocorticoids, or other conditions that cause increased bone loss.

Findings

Radiographic lucency(after 30% of bone mineral is lost)
Bone density >2.5 standard deviations (SDs) below the young adult mean value (T-score <−2.5)*

*T-score <−1 to −2.5 is termed 'osteopenia'.
What are the treatment strategies?

Big Head. . .

For the ensuing weeks Irene's diagnosis of osteoporosis was the main topic of discussion.' Your bones are thinning out dear' John remarked. He then went on to talk about 'Big Head', one of the regulars at the pub. 'I think Big Head has the opposite problem'. John said. 'His bones are growing, getting very thick. He'll have to change his hat soon.' Big Head could be suffering from Paget's disease.

Trigger box   Paget's disease

Excessive osteoclast resorption and disorganized osteoblastic activity causing abnormal and weak new bone.

15% involving one bone (monostotic), 85% polyostotic.

Common sites in order of frequency: pelvis, lumbar spine, femur, thoracic spine, sacrum, skull, tibia.

Genetic disposition. Chromosome 18q.

Positive family history 14%.

Men: women ratio = 2:3.

More in Europeans.

Most are asymptomatic.

Features: Bone pain, joint pain, deformities (e.g. skull enlargement and bowed legs) and fractures due to the new softer woven bones, nerve compression.

Increased bone blood flow (myocardial hypertrophy and high-output heart failure).

Osteogenic sarcoma (rare <1% but a 30% increased risk).

Findings: X-ray: lytic lesions, sclerotic lesions.

Bone scan: can show extent of disease.

Raised alkaline phosphatase.

Treatment: Bisphosphonates.

Jane's hot joints. . .

Jane, Mary's sister was staying with Irene at this time. She had come to visit the Sickalotts after her husband had suddenly left her some 6 months ago. A few months after Irene's accident and the subsequent diagnosis of osteoporosis, Jane mentioned her joint problems. Her hand joints were poorly, she said. She complained that they were stiff, swollen and tender. She had also noticed a bump over her small finger in her right hand. In addition to her hands Jane also had swelling in her right and left knees and complained of dry eyes and mouth. Mary took her to see Dr Smith.

Dr Smith took a history. Jane's symptoms were worse in the mornings but got better as the day progressed. She suffered from intermittent feverishness, malaise, and had lost weight.

Table 6.7 Jane's laboratory findings

Haemoglobin	119 g/L (115–160)
WCC	14.6×10^9 (4–11)
Platelets	460 (150–400)
Neutrophils	10.8(2–7.5)
Monocytes	1.4 (00–1.00)
ESR	60 mm/H (0–20)
CRP	25 mg/L (0–10)
RF titre	250 (0–30)
LFTs	Normal
U & Es	Normal
ANA	Positive

ANA, antinuclear antibody; CRP, C-reactive protein; ESR, erythrocyte sedimentation rate.

He examined her. Her vitals were normal. Jane's proximal interphalangeal joints were swollen and tender for several fingers in both hands. Her distal IP joints were not affected. There were small effusions in both knees. He also noted conjunctivitis and a dry mouth. Dr Smith took some blood for lab tests: the results are shown in Table 6.7.

Can you explain these results?

What does the increase in ESR and CRP suggest?

What is rheumatoid factor (RF)?

He prescribed artificial tears for her dry eyes and referred her to a rheumatologist, Dr Green. 'I'm afraid you may be suffering from rheumatoid arthritis' he said.

What are the differences in the hand pathology in rheumatoid and osteoarthritis?

Dr Green confirmed Dr Smith's diagnosis. He aspirated some joint fluid which showed a yellow fluid with leucocytes and fibrin strands

Can you interpret the synovial fluid findings?

Dr Green explained the nature of Jane's condition. He explained the autoimmune basis of the disease and went over its systemic features. He particularly mentioned Sjogrens syndrome, which accounted for her dry eyes and mouth.

Trigger box   Rheumatoid arthritis

Synovial disease, infiltration of chronic inflammatory cells, cytokines (e.g. TNF-α, IL 8).

Synovium becomes pannus, which destroys cartilage and bone.

Aetiology unknown.

Women:men ratio $= 3:1$.

Any age but usually 30 to 50 years old.

Types

1. **Articular**

   70% of cases. Slowly progressive, symmetrical, peripheral polyarthritis, evolving over weeks or months.

   15% of cases: Rapid onset, severe.

   Usually pain and stiffness of small joints of the hands (MCP, PIP joints), feet (MTP).

   Morning stiffness, pain, feeling tired and unwell. Improves with gentle activity. Affected joints are warm, tender with some joint swelling. Muscle wasting, limitation of movement and deformities in later stages syndrome.

   Usually many joints affected: wrists, elbows, shoulders, knees and ankles. Ten per cent monarthritis of the knee or shoulder or carpal tunnel. Hips rarely affected in early stages.

2. **Non-articular**

   Subcutaneous nodules. Peripheral and intrapulmonary nodules. Caplan's syndrome (large cavitating lung nodules in co-existing pneumoconiosis).

   Serositis causing pleural effusion, fibrosing alveolitis, obstructive bronchiolitis.

   Vasculitis.

   Rarely pericarditis, endocarditis and myocardial diseases.

   Raynaud's syndrome.

   Neuropathies due to mononeuritis multiplex, compression (carpal or tarsal tunnel syndrome). Atlanto-axial subluxation can cause serious neurological damages.

   Scleritis, episcleritis.

   Sjögren's syndrome (causing dry mouth and eyes).

   Amyloidosis causing nephrotic syndrome and renal failure.

   Splenomegaly and neutropenia (Felty's syndrome).

   Anaemia of chronic disease.

   Haemolytic anaemia (Coombs' positives). Pancytopenia due to hypersplenism (Felty's syndrome) or DMARD treatment.

   Findings: Pannus; IgM rheumatoid factor(RF) in 70%(RF associated with aggressive disease), nodules; anti-nuclear antibody (ANA) in 30%; Normochromic normocytic anaemia. Thrombocytopenia (associated with active disease).

   Raised ESR, CRP.

   Poorer prognosis factors are female, gradual onset over a few months, positive IgM rheumatoid factor, developing anaemia within 3 months of onset.

What are the features of Sjögren's syndrome

Jane was positive for rheumatoid factor and ANA, two diagnostically important autoantibodies. Other key autoantibodies and their associated diseases are shown in Table 6.8.

Dr Green prescribed indometacin (NSAID) and preclnisolone. He also mentioned that he might have to give her methotrexate, a disease-modifying anti-rheumatic drug (DMARD).Jane was also referred for physiotherapy. Figure 6.12 shows the arachidonic acid pathway and indicates where COX 1 and COX 2 inhibitors work. Table 6.9 shows the medications used in RA.

Table 6.8 Autoantibodies and their associated diseases

Autoantibody	Disease
ANA, anti Ds DNA, anti-cardiolipin, RF	SLE
Anti-adrenal gland	Addison's disease
Anti-Lo, Anti La	Sjögren's disease
Anti-IgG (IgM antibody-RF), ANA	RA
Anti-histone	SLE (drug induced)
Anti-Scl-70	Diffuse scleroderma
Anti-centromere	CREST
C ANCA	Wegener's granulomatosis
P ANCA	PAN, microscopic polyangiitis
Anti-mitochondrial	Primary biliary cirrhosis
Anti-endomyseal ⎫	Coeliac disease
Anti-TTG　　　　⎬	
Anti-gliadin 　　⎭	
Anti-epithelial	Pemphigus vulgaris
Anti-microsomal, anti-thyroglobulin	Graves' disease
Anti-microsomal	Hashimoto's thyroiditis
Anti-basement membrane	Goodpasture's syndrome
Anti-red cell	Cold haemolytic anaemia
Anti-AchR	Myasthenia gravis
Anti-gastric parietal cell antibodies (AGPCAs) and anti intrinsic factor antibodies (IF Abs).	Pernicious anaemia
Anti-smooth muscle	Chronic active hepatitis
Anti-smooth muscle, ANA	Autoimmune hepatitis
Anti-MPO-ANCA	Primary sclerosing cholangitis
Anti-platelet	ITP
Anti Jo-1	Polymyositis and dermatomyositis

  Compare and contrast osteo and rheumatoid arthritis.

Trigger box   **Juvenile rheumatoid arthritis (JRA)**

<16 years, most settle by puberty.

Features: Fever (daily, high spiking), nodules, fatigue, pericarditis, salmon rash, hepatosplenomegaly, serositis.

Types:

1. *Pauciarticular JRA*: Affecting ≤ 4 joints. Most common form. 30% develop iridiocyclitis. ANA, RF (in ankylosing spondylitis males).
2. *Polyarticular JRA* :≥ 5 joints. Multiple, symmetrical small joints.
3. *Systemic onset JRA*: with high fever, rash.

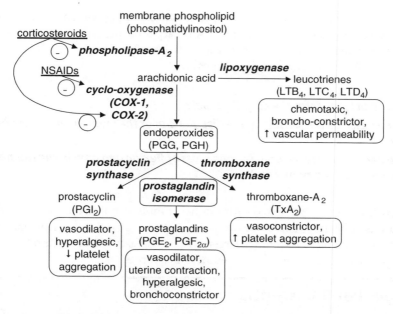

Figure 6.12 Arachidonic acid metabolism showing sites of key anti-inflammatory drug action. Adapted from Rang, Dale, Ritter, and Moore (2003) Pharmacolgy, 5th edition, Churchill Livingstone

Some 4 months later Jane was back in Dr Green's clinic. Her right hand had become painful and she had pins and needles, which were waking her from sleep. She complained of loss of flexion and pain in the thumb and index finger of the right hand, which has been increasing gradually over the previous four months, Dr Green found that there was numbness over the first three fingers and the radial half of the ring finger. She had taken extra NSAIDs but the condition had not improved.

Table 6.9 Drugs used in the treatment of rheumatoid arthritis

1. Paracetamol and NSAIDs: for pain relief. (e.g. ibuprofen, diclofenac).

2. Steroids: to control flare-ups. (e.g. oral prednisolone, intra-articular injections with semicrystalline steroids, intramuscular depo injections).

3. Disease-modifying anti-rheumatic drugs (DMARDs): control symptoms and slow structural damage (e.g. sulfasalazine, methotrexate, sodium aurothiomalate, leflunamide, hydroxychloroquine, D-penicillamine and less commonly azathioprine, ciclosporin).

4. Biological therapies: Halt or reverse bone erosion. Inhibit progression of radiographic joint damage. TNF-α blockers (e.g. adalimumab, infliximab, etanercept), Recombinant human antagonist of interleukin 1 (IL-1) (e.g. anakinra).

Dr Green carried out EMG and nerve conduction studies, which showed decreased median nerve conduction. The diagnosis was carpal tunnel syndrome. X-ray analysis showed narrowing of joint spaces between carpal bones.

Jane was referred for surgical decompression.

Which structures form the carpal tunnel?

Can you describe the sensory nerve distribution of the median, ulnar and radial nerve?

Which nerve damage resulted in Jane's loss of flexion and pain in the thumb and index finger of the right hand?

A few years later Jane presented with another complication: an ulcer on her right shin. The area was ischaemic. There was distal symmetrical sensorimotor neuropathy and a nodule on the Achilles tendon. Dr Green suspected vascultis. He reminded Jane that vascultis was a complication of her rheumatoid arthritis.

Trigger box Vasculitis

1. *Large vessels (aorta & main vessels)*
   E.g.: **Takayasu's arteritis:** pulseless, raised ESR, more common in Asians, arthritis, myalgia, skin nodules.

2. *Medium vessels (visceral, coronary, renal)*
   Examples
   Polyarteritis nodosa (PAN): pANCA, hepatitisB, immune complexes, pericarditis, myocarditis.
   Kawasaki disease: Children especially Japanese & Korean; conjunctivitis, rash, adenopathy, strawberry tongue, fever, oedema, coronary artery aneurysms, MI.
   Temporal arteritis: Carotid branches; headaches, jaw claudication, polymyalgia rheumatica (PMR) (50%), high ESR.

3. *Small vessels (arterioles, venules, capillaries)*
   Examples
   Microscopic polyangitis: pANCA; focal segmental glomerulonephritis.
   Wegener's granulomatosis: cANCA, nasal, lung.
   Churg–Strauss syndrome: Asthma, eosinophilia, systemic vasculitis.
   Henoch–Schönlein purpura: Children, purpura, IgA immune complexes, arthritis, nephritis.

How do you treat these conditions?

What are the main features of polymyalgia rheumatica?

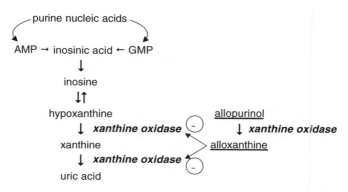

Figure 6.13   Nucleic acid metabolism and gout. Adapted from Stryer (1988), Biochemistry, 3rd edition, Freeman

John and his hot, red, big toe...

One day John woke up with severe pain in his left toe. Switching the light on he noticed that his toe was red and swollen. The next day he went off to see Dr Smith who diagnosed gouty arthritis. He was prescribed indometacin. The relevant metabolic pathway is shown in Fig. 6.13.

 What is the pathophysiology of gout? Why do individuals who eat lots of red meat and wine more likely to develop gout?

Trigger box   Gout

M>F.

Pathology: Monosodium urate crystals (negatively birefringent) in joint.

Findings: Hyperuricaemia.

Causes: Decreased excretion of uric acid, G6PD deficiency, Lesh–Nyhan syndrome, phosphyoribosylribophosphate (PRPP) excess, thiazides.

Features: Podagra, tophi.

Treatment: Allopurinol, colchicine, NSAIDs, probenecid.

7

The nervous system

Learning strategy

In this chapter we will consider the essential, 'must know' facts and concepts of the nervous system. Our main strategy will involve an exploration of these key principles via the clinical examination of the nervous system.

A carpal tunnel injury will introduce you to neuronal anatomy and physiology. The anatomy and physiology of the central nervous system will be covered through a stroke scenario where loss of function will highlight key brain regions and their functions.

A scenario involving Parkinson's disease will introduce you to neurotransmitters and synaptic transmission. A meningitis scare will introduce the meninges and cerebrospinal fluid (CSF).

Testing the integrity of the vagus nerve will lead us to consider the autonomic nervous system. This will lead us to the key drugs modulating the nervous system.

Throughout, we will also consider the pathophysiological mechanisms of several common diseases, which will, in addition to highlighting the key pathophysiological principles, further reinforce basic principles of neuroanatomy, physiology and pharmacology.

Try to answer the questions and complete the Learning Tasks.

Jane's carpal tunnel

Jane's wrist problem was getting worse. Her rheumatoid arthritis was up and down but more than anything her right wrist was concerning her. She had sensations of

Integrated Medical Sciences by Shantha Perera, Stephen Anderson, Ho Leung and Rousseau Gama
© 2007 John Wiley & Sons, Ltd ISBN: 978470016589 (HB) 978470016596 (PB)

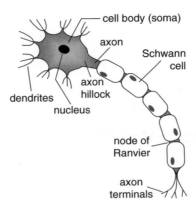

Figure 7.1   Neuron structure

pins and needles and her hand was often painful. Often at night she was woken up by the pain; she found dangling her hand over the bed and giving it a vigorous shake often helpful.

   Review the sensory distribution of the radial, ulnar and median nerves. A good way to remember this is to paint your hand!

Jane's nerve conduction defect can be used to introduce the basic unit of the nervous system, the neuron. The basic structure of the neuron is illustrated in Figure 7.1

Apart from the neuron there are other cells which constitute the nervous system. Table 7.1 shows the different types of accessory cell found in the nervous system.

Now, these cells can become cancerous giving rise to the various CNS tumours. Key information about these cancers is shown in Table 7.2.

   What are the cancers that metastasize to the brain? Do brain tumours metastasize to the rest of the body?

Table 7.1   Types of accessory cell in the nervous system

Cell	Function
Microglial cell	Phagocyte
Oligodendroglial cell	Myelinates CNS axons
Schwann cell	Myelinates PNS cells
Astrocyte	Facilitates exchange between capillaries & neurones
Ependymal cells	Line ventricles; helps circulation of CSF

PNS, peripheral nervous system.

Table 7.2   CNS tumours

Tumour type	Main features
Astrocytoma	Increased intracranial pressure (ICP), headache (HA), cranial nerve (CN) palsies, slow course. Treatment: resection/radiation
GBM (grade IV astrocytoma)	Most common primary brain tumour Rapid progression, death <1 year Treatment: Radiation, resection, chemotherapy
Meningioma	Dura/arachnoid tumour Prognosis good Treatment: Surgery, radiation
Schwannoma (acoustic neuroma)	Schwann cell tumour Ipsilateral hearing loss, tinnitus, vertigo Treatment: Surgery
Medulloblastoma	Arises from the 4th ventricle: primitive neuroectodermal cell Causes increased ICP Very malignant Common in children Treatment: Surgery, radiation, chemotherapy
Ependymoma	Causes hydrocephalus Common in children Treatment: Surgery, radiation

GBM: Glioblastoma multiforme

We can now turn to the conduction of nerve impulses, the primary function of a neuron. In Jane's case nerve conduction studies demonstrated slowing of conduction of the median nerve.

Figure 7.2 shows how a typical neuron responds to a stimulus. Note the resting membrane potential, the threshold potentials, depolarization, repolarization and the refractory periods. The mechanisms propagating the action potential are depicted in Figure 7.3.

 Describe the 'All or Nothing' phenomenon of action potentials observed in neurons.

Jane's median nerve is composed of a large number of axons. The electrical activity recorded is a *total* of all the individual action potentials in all the neurons that make up the nerve. This is the compound action potential.

Nerve conduction velocity is determined by: (1) axon diameter and (2) myelination. Nerve conduction is *increased* by axon diameter and myelination.

 How is the nerve impulse propagated along a myelinated neuron?

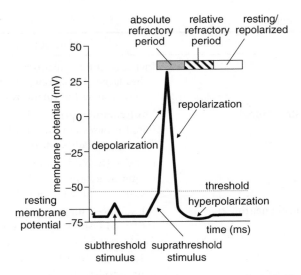

Figure 7.2 Neuron action potentials. Adapted from McGeown (1999) Physiology, Churchill Livingstone

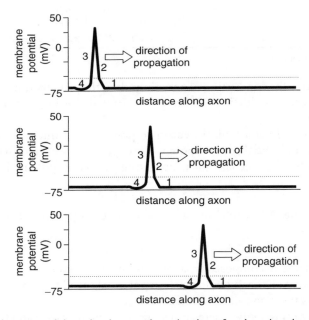

Figure 7.3 Action potential mechanisms and conduction of an impulse along an axon. 1. Na$^+$ channels in resting state, K$^+$ channels closed. 2. Na$^+$ channels open. 3. K$^+$ channels open, Na$^+$ channels inactivated. 4. Hyperpolarization (K$^+$ channels open, Na$^+$ channels resting). Adapted from McGeown (1999) Physiology, Churchill Livingstone

Trigger box **Multiple sclerosis**

Multiple demyelinations within brain and spinal cord (optic nerves, periventricular regions, brainstem, cerebellum, C spinal cord (corticospinal tracts and posterior columns). Female > male, early adulthood, rare in tropics.
Findings: Optic nerve inflammation – blurred vision/unilateral eye pain.
Optic neuritis and atrophy, diplopia, vertigo, dysphagia, nystagmus, paraesthesia, spastic paraparesis.
Investigations: MRI, evoked potentials (prolonged), CSF (WBC, IgG raised, oligoclonal bands).
Treatment: Steroids, interferon-β (reduces relapse rate), physiotherapy natalizumab.

Find out about the different *patterns* of MS.

What are evoked potentials?

Trigger box **Guillain–Barré syndrome (acute postinfective polyneuropathy)**

Acute inflammatory demyelinating polyneuropathy.
CMI response against peripheral myelin.
Campylobacter jejuni, cytomegalovirus (CMV) infection can precede.
Findings: Progressive distal muscle weakness, numbness and areflexia, respiratory muscles involved.
Investigations: Nerve conduction studies, CSF protein (elevated).
Monitor vital capacity, ECG.
Treatment: Intravenous gamma-globulin, plasmapheresis, heparin (to reduce venous thrombosis risk), physiotherapy.

Albert's tremor . . .

For some months now, Albert had noticed that his hands were trembling. He was quite distressed about this especially because he was finding it difficult to dress himself and carry out his everyday tasks. He decided to visit the Surgery. Maybe Dr Smith can give me some medicine to control it, he thought. . .

Dr Smith enquired about the tremor. It was present most of the time; even when Albert was resting but seemed to disappear when he was using his hands.

The tremor was classically of the 'pill rolling' type. On examination he also noted some cogwheel rigidity – an increased muscle tone and resistance to passive movement. He also noted a decrease in Albert's facial expression The diagnosis was clear: Albert was showing signs of Parkinson's disease (PD).

 Describe the different types of tremor stating their likely causes.

Trigger box   **Parkinson's disease (PD)**

Extrapyramidal disorder.
Depletion of dopamine containing neurons in substantia nigra of basal ganglia.
1:200 over 70.
Causes: Idiopathic mainly, MPTP (methylphenyltetrahydropyridine).
Findings: Tremor: rigidity (lead pipe, cogwheel) akinesia, dysphagia, micrographia, excess acetylcholine.
Treatment: Levodopa is the mainstay of therapy.
(Use with a depo-decarboxylase inhibitor e.g. carbidopa, to give a dose-sparing effect by reducing peripheral metabolic inactivation.)
Other drugs: bromocriptine, selegiline, amantadine, anticholinergics (what are their MOAs?).
On–off syndrome with medication.
Surgery: Stereotactic thalamotomy or pallidotomy in patients where severe tremor or dyskinesia not responsive to therapeutic intervention.

Albert is likely to eventually show symptoms of dementia as PD patients can suffer from dementia.

Trigger box   **Dementia**

Higher cortical functions disturbed.
Consciousness *not* clouded.
10% over 65; 20% over 80.
Most common cause: Alzheimer's disease.
Other causes: strokes, Wernicke–Korsakoff syndrome, hypothyroidism, vitamin B_{12} deficiency, syphilis, Creutzfeldt–Jakob disease (CJD), Huntington's disease, Parkinson's disease, chronic trauma, hydrocephalus, haematoma.
Average survival 9 years.

Alzheimer's disease
Unknown aetiology.
Features: Slow progression, short-term memory loss, personality changes, intellect loss. Neurofibrillary tangles, amyloid plaques in brain.
Investigations: Mental state assessment, CT, vitamin B_{12} and folate levels, LFT, TFT, FBC.
Treatment: Donepezil (acetylcholine esterase inhibitors).

Albert's Parkinsonism was due to a decrease in the neurotransmitter dopamine. This gives us an opportunity to consider synaptic transmission and the important role of neurotransmitters in the propagation of the nerve impulse from one neuron to the next.

Figure 7.4 shows what happens at a synapse. As seen, synaptic transmission involves the release of neurotransmitters, which either stimulate or inhibit action potentials in

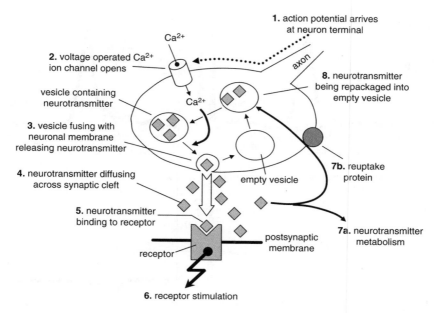

Figure 7.4 Synaptic transmission. Adapted from Rang, Dale, Ritter and Moore (2003) Pharmacology, 5th edition, Churchill Livingstone

the postsynaptic neuron. Table 7.3 shows the key neurotransmitters. Complete Table 7.3.

Excitatory neurotransmitters like acetylcholine and glutamate cause depolarization of the postsynaptic membrane. The response in the postsynaptic neurone is called the

Table 7.3 Key neurotransmitters complete table

Transmitter	Receptor	Receptor locations
Acetylcholine (ACh)	Nicotinic	Neuromuscular junction, autonomic ganglia, CNS.
	Muscarinic	Tissues innervated by PNS, CNS
Noradrenaline (NA)	α_{1+2} and β_{1-3}	Tissues innervated by the SNS, CNS
5-hydroxytryptamine (5-HT, serotonin)	5-HT_{1-7}	Gastrointestinal tract, platelets, CNS.
Dopamine (DA)	D_{1-5}	CNS.
Histamine	H_{1-3}	CNS as neurotransmitter receptors, but also occur in periphery as autacoid receptors
Glycine	- - - - -	- - - - -
Glutamate	- - - - -	- - - - -
Gamma-aminobutyric acid (GABA)	GABA_{A+B}	CNS

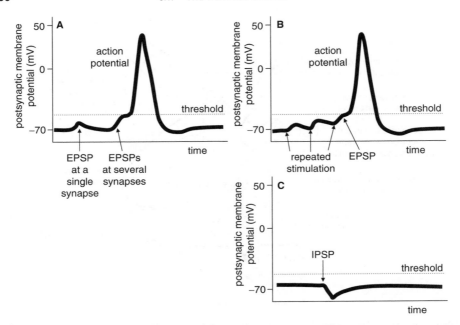

Figure 7.5 Excitatory postsynaptic potential (EPSP): spatial summation (A) and temporal summation (B) produced in response to excitatory transmitters e.g., glutamate. (C) Inhibitory postsynaptic potential (IPSP) produced in response to inhibitory transmitters, e.g. glycine. Adapted from McGeown (1999) Physiology, Churchill Livingstone

excitatory postsynaptic potential (EPSP). Features of the EPSP, such as spatial and temporal summation are shown in Figure 7.5.

Similarly, inhibitory neurotransmitters like glycine and GABA cause hyperpolarization in the postsynaptic membrane. This is called the inhibitory postsynaptic potential (IPSP) (Figure 7.5). IPSPs and EPSPs summate algebraically.

The magnitude of the EPSP can be also reduced by the action of inhibitory nerves which act presynaptically to inhibit the presynaptic cell, hence reducing the amount of neurotransmitter released at the synapse. Examples are inhibitory interneurons found in the spinal cord.

Albert was eventually treated with levadopa which markedly improved his symptoms. Levadopa increased the amount of dopamine. The MOA of levadopa is shown in Figure 7.6.

Table 7.4 shows the main disorders where fluctuations of neurotransmitters are thought to be responsible for many of the symptoms of the diseases.

Drugs used in the treatment of schizophrenia can cause development of Parkinsonian symptoms. Can you explain the mechanism underlying this observation?

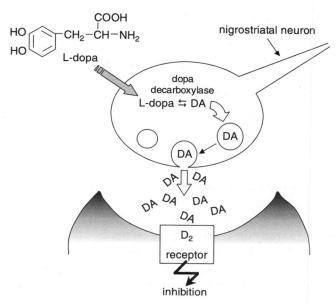

Figure 7.6 Conversion of levadopa (L-dopa) into dopamine (DA). Adapted from Rang, Dale, Ritter and Moore (2003) Pharmacology, 5th edition, Churchill Livingstone

Table 7.4 Neurotransmitters and disease

Disease	Neurotransmitter defect(s)	Treatment examples
Depression	↓NE, ↓5HT	Fluoxetine, Phenelzine
Anxiety	↑NE, ↓GABA, ↓5HT	Diazepam
Alzheimer's Disease	↓Ach	Artane, Cogentin
Huntington's Disease	↓GABA, ↓Ach	
Schizophrenia	↑dopamine	Haloperidol
Parkinson's disease	↓dopamine	Carbidopa

ACh, acetylcholine, NE, noradrenaline, GABA, gammaaminobutyric acid, 5HT 5 hydroxytryptamine

 Can you work out the rationale of the treatment strategies?

Now that we have considered the basic structure and functioning of the neuron we can turn to the overall organization of the nervous system a simple classification of which is shown in Figure 7.7 below. Note that the vagus (a cranial nerve) has autonomic functions.

What are the components that make up a nerve like the median nerve? Draw a cross-sectional diagram and label the key structures?

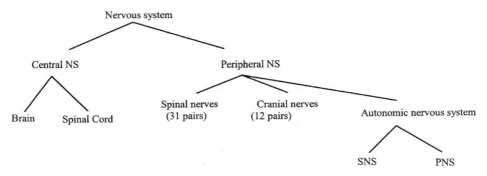

Figure 7.7 Classification of the nervous system

We are now ready to study the central nervous system.

The main structural and functional features of the central nervous system are best illustrated by looking at what happens when an insult leads to loss of function. This can be illustrated by describing what happened to Irene one winters' evening.

A bad night for Irene . . .

Albert woke up startled: Irene had woken up and was moving about in bed. She looked agitated. She appeared confused and was trying to say something, but wasn't able to speak coherently. Frightened, Albert called Mary. Mary arrived a few minutes later and immediately called for the ambulance.

The paramedics arrived 10 minutes later. Irene was still incoherent. The senior paramedic immediately noted signs of a right-sided hemiparesis: he asked Irene to grasp his index and middle fingers with her hands and noted reduced power in her right hand. Irene was taken to the ED at Hope Hospital.

Irene had suffered from a stroke. Later on it was established that she had suffered from a thrombotic stroke where a thrombus had blocked one of her cranial blood vessels.

Trigger box Stroke

Incidence 1.5/1000; rising to 10/1000 at 75 years.
Third most common cause of death in UK.
Patients generally over 40 years.
Focal neurological deficit lasting >24 h.
Completed stroke by 6 h.
Transient ischaemic attack (TIA) <24 h; complete recovery.

Causes:

1. *Cerebral infarction* (85%): caused by thrombosis, emboli (e.g. from post- MI, AFib), severe HTN. Cerebral hemisphere infarct 50% (commonest cause of hemiplegia), lacunar infarction 25%, brainstem infarct 25%.

2. *Cerebral haemorrhage* (15%): e.g. ruptured aneurysms.

   Findings: Severe headaches, vomiting, coma, neurological deficits, initial hypotonia then spastic hemiplegia, lateral medullary syndrome (in brainstem infarct).
   Investigation: CT/MRI, blood glucose, U & E, ECG.
   Treatment: For cerebral infarct (after exclusion of intracranial haemorrhage): aspirin, thrombolytics, heparin.
   25% die within 2 years.

The thrombus in one of Irene's arteries supplying the brain allows us to consider the blood supply to the brain. Figure 7.8 shows the main blood supply to the brain.

Table 7.5 shows the brain regions supplied from the circle of Willis. Complete Table 7.5.

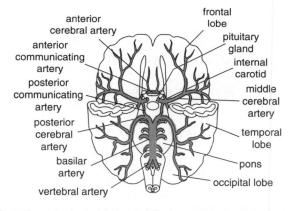

Figure 7.8   Blood supply to the brain/circle of Willis (ventral regions of temporal lobes removed for clarity). Adapted from Marieb (1995) Human Anatomy and Physiology, 3rd edition, Benjamin Cummings

Table 7.5   Brain regions supplied by the circle of Willis

Artery	Brain region supplied	Functions/Lesions
Anterior cerebral artery	Medial brain	Motor/sensory cortex (leg, foot area)
Middle cerebral artery	- - - - - -	- - - - - -
Anterior communicating artery	- - - - - -	Visual field defects
Posterior communicating artery	- - - - - -	CN III palsies
Lateral striae	- - - - - -	- - - - - -

What do we mean by the blood–brain barrier? Describe the structures forming the blood–brain barrier?

Strokes can also be haemorrhagic. Haemorrhagic strokes can be caused by intracerebral, subarachnoid, subdural or extradural (epidural) haemorrhages.

Trigger box   Intracranial haemorrhages

1. *Intracerebral*
   More common in elderly.
   Within brain parenchyma.
   Causes: HTN, tumour, amyloid, arteriovenous malformation (AVM).
   Features: Lethargy, headache, focal neurological signs.
   Investigations: CT.
   Treatment: see SAH.

2. *Subarachnoid* (SAH)
   Much less common.
   Incidence 15/100 000, typical age 35–65 years
   Causes: Ruptured berry aneurysms, congenital AVM.
   Features: Severe immediate headache, third nerve palsy, subhyaloid haemorrhage, loss of consciousness (LOC), N & V, meningeal signs.
   The headache in SAH is often described by patients as 'the worst headache in my life'.
   Investigations: CT, LP (xanthochromia)
   Treatment: Surgery to clip off aneurysm, dexamethasone, nimodipine (for vasospasm).
   50% immediate mortality.

3. *Subdural*
   Venous bleed.
   Causes: Head injury.
   Features: Symptoms weeks and months from injury, headache, confusion, drowsiness.
   Investigations: CT.
   Treatment: Surgery (evacuation of haematoma via burr holes).

4. *Epidural* (extradural)
   Causes: Head injury. Temporal bone fracture – middle meningeal artery.
   Features: LOC followed by lucid interval then rapid deterioration with focal signs.
   Investigations: CT.
   Treatment: Surgery (urgent evacuation of clot via multiple burr holes and then identification and ligation of bleeding vessels).

Trigger box **Headaches**

1. *Migraine*
   Female > male.
   Family history.
   Putative pathogenesis: Vascular, serotonin abnormalities.
   Triggers (e.g. cheese, chocolate).
   Features: Unilateral, throbbing, nausea & vomiting, photophobia, visual aura (classic migraine); bilateral, periorbital (common migraines).
   Treatment: Avoid triggers, $5HT_1$ agonists (triptans), NSAIDs.
   Prophylaxis: Beta-blockers, amitriptyline, sodium valproate, calcium channel blockers.

2. *Cluster headache*
   Male > female, average onset 25.
   Features: Unilateral, periorbital, up to 3 h, same time same place.
   Ipsilateral tearing pain, transient ipsilateral Horner's syndrome common.
   Treatment: Triptans, inhalation of O_2.

3. *Tension headache*
   Most common type. Tension within scalp muscles.
   Features: Tight band like, occipital/neck pain, no focal neurological signs
   Treatment: Reassurance, relaxation, massage, check refractive errors.

The CNS is covered by the meninges. We can consider the meninges by looking at what happened (or didn't happen) to Little John when he was 3.

Little John's rash...

Little John developed a rash after suffering from a cold for 3 days. He was miserable, was feeding poorly and had a high fever. Mary became worried. 'What if it is meningitis?' she thought. A visit to see Dr Smith, however, allayed her fears. 'This is a typical viral rash' Dr Smith said. Just for thoroughness he tested for photophobia and neck stiffness the absence of which pretty much ruled out meningitis. Figure 7.9 shows the meninges and the formation and flow of CSF.

> Describe how you would elicit Kernig's and Brudzinski's signs.

> Blockage of the flow of CSF can give rise to hydrocephalus. Describe communicating and non-communicating types of hydrocephalus.

If Little John was suspected of having meningitis a lumbar puncture would be performed to examine CSF. A typical analysis is shown in Table 7.6.

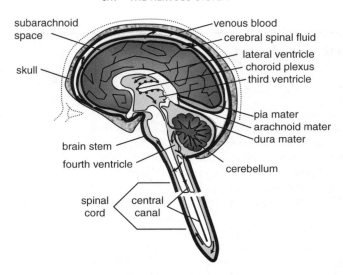

Figure 7.9 The meninges and the formation and flow of CSF

Table 7.6 Meningitis: analysis of CSF

	Pressure	Cell type	Protein	Glucose
Bacteria	↑↑	PMN	↑↑ (>100 mg/dL)	↓↓ (<45 mg/dL)
Fungal/TB	↑↑	Lymphocyte	↑↑(50–100 mg/dL)	↓↓ (<45 mg/dL)
Viral	N/↑	Lymphocyte	N (15–45mg/dL)	N (45–85 mg/dL)
Normal	N	–	15–45 mg/dL	45–85 mg/dL

N, no change;

Trigger box   Meningitis

Findings: Rapid onset severe headache, photophobia, vomiting, malaise, fever, Kernig's & Brudzinski's signs, petechiae, papilloedema.
Fulminant meningococcal meningitis – large eccymoses, gangrene.
Consciousness intact but may be delirious with fever. Progressive drowsiness with complications.
Bacterial causes of meningitis

1. *Newborn*
   Streptococcus Group B, *Escherichia coli*, *Listeria monocytogenes*

2. *Children (6 months–6 years)*
   Streptococcus pneumoniae, Neisseria meningitidis, Haemophilus influenzae b,

3. *Young children, adolescents, young adults*
   Neisseria meningitidis

4. *Adults (including elderly)*
   Streptococcus pneumoniae.

   Transmission: Respiratory, direct spread from otitis media, skull fracture, sinusitis.
   Viral meningitis – benign, self-limiting.
   Investigations: LP.
   Treatment: Immediate i.v. benzylpenicillin, cefotaxime.
   Complications: hyponatraemia, seizures, subdural effusions, brain abscess, ventriculi-
   tis, subdural empyema.
   Mortality may be 30%. (bacterial meningitis)

Trigger box   **Encephalitis**

Inflammation of the brain.
Pathogens: Arboviruses, herpes simplex virus (HSV, causes severe disease), HIV.
Children mainly.
Findings: Headache, drowsiness, fever, neck stiffness, confusion, stupor, coma.
Hemiparesis, positive Babinski's sign, increased deep tendon reflexes (DTR), seizures,
diabetes insipidus.
Raised ICP causes papilloedema and CN III, CN VI palsies.
Investigations: CT, LP (CSF shows mononucleosis, and increased protein).
Treatment: HSV – aciclovir; CMV – ganciclovir and foscarnet.

The LP procedure allows us to turn to the anatomy of the spinal cord. Figure 7.10 shows
the main features of the spinal cord.

Note the sensory and motor pathways, which we will consider later.

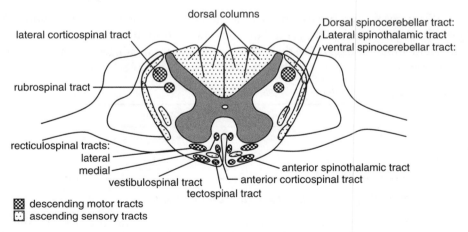

Figure 7.10 Location of sensory and motor tracts within the spinal cord. Adapted from Tortora
and Grabowski (2003), Principles of Anatomy and Physiology, 10th edition, John Wiley & Sons

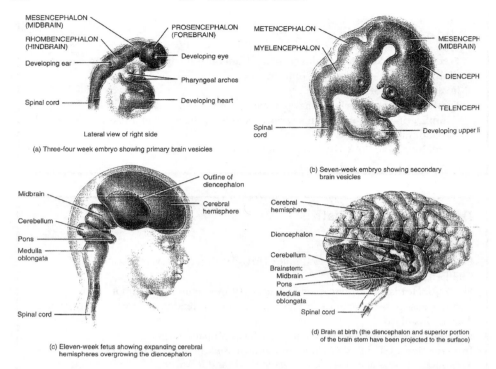

Figure 7.11   Development of the central nervous system. Adapted from Tortora and Grabowski (2003), Principles of Anatomy and Physiology, 10th Edition, John Wiley and Sons Inc. New York

What are the structures pierced in turn by the needle during the lumbar puncture? Where do you position the needle?

To which vertebral level does the spinal cord reach in the newborn and in the adult?

At this point we can briefly review how the nervous system develops. Figure 7.11 shows the development of the central nervous system from the neural tube.

In neural tube defects (NTDs) the spinal cord and/or the meninges herniate through a pathological opening in the vertebral column. Complete Table 7.7 on NTDs

Table 7.7   Neural tube defects

Type	Pathology	Features	Management
Spina bifida occulta	- - - - - - - -	- - - - - - - -	- - - - - - - -
Meningocele	- - - - - - - -	- - - - - - - -	- - - - - - - -
Meningomyelocele	- - - - - - - -	- - - - - - - -	- - - - - - - -

What should pregnant women take to prevent NTDs

Let us return to Irene. At the hospital Irene was a bit more communicative. Her speech had improved sufficiently to converse with the doctor. She mentioned that her right side felt 'strange'.

She mentioned having a few 'funny turns' over the past couple of months. The doctor also spoke to Mary and obtained more details of Irene's medical history.

Irene's 'funny turns' could have been transient ischaemic attacks (TIAs). What are the key features of TIAs?

The doctor then began his examination. She was afebrile; her BP was 175/102, her pulse 97 and regular.

He noted that her speech was slurred but her comprehension appeared normal. He asked her name, present location, and date. He asked her to name an object – his pen, and asked her to point at a named object – the calendar on the wall. She answered his questions correctly. He asked her to say 'British Constitution' and he noticed that her speech was impaired.

Let us now consider what the doctor was testing. He was carrying out a quick examination of her 'higher' functions. Which parts of the brain are responsible for these higher functions? What are the functions of the other key regions of the brain? What are the functional consequences of damage to these different regions? Table 7.8 shows the key functions of the lobes of the brain. Fig 7.12 shows the basic anatomy of the brain.

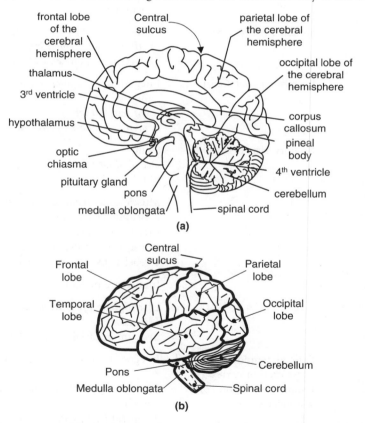

Figure 7.12 Anatomy of the brain. Adapted from Tortora, (2003), A Photographic Atlas of the Human Body, Second Edition, John Wiley and Sons

Table 7.8   The functions of the lobes of the brain (see Figure 7.12)

Lobe	Area	Function/some examples of lesion effects
Frontal	Prefrontal association cortex	Personality traits, decision making, voluntary activity planning. *Frontal lobe lesions:* Personality changes, dementia, amnesia, loss of executive functions. *Dominant frontal lobe lesions:* Expressive aphasia.
	Premotor cortex	Movement coordination.
	Supplementary motor area	Complex movement programming.
	Primary motor cortex	Voluntary movement. *Primary motor cortex lesions:* Hemiplegia (also lesions in descending motor tracts, internal capsule can cause hemiplegia).
Parietal	Somatosensory cortex	Somatic sensation and proprioception. *Cortical sensory region lesions.* Contralateral hemianaesthesia.
	Posterior parietal cortex	Integration of somatosensory and visual inputs. *Right parietal lobe lesions.* Spatial awareness disorders, neglect.
Occipital	Primary visual cortex	Sight. *Occipital lobe lesions:* Blindness.
Cerebellum		Muscle tone, balance, synchronization of muscle activity. *Cerebellar lesions:* ataxia, nystagmus, ocular dysmetria, cerebellar tremor, dysarthria.
Hippocampus:		Immediate memory.
Brain stem		Disconguate eye movements, *Lesions:* nystagmus, facial palsies, ataxia.
Temporal	Parietal–temporal–occipital association cortex	Integration of sensory input, language.
	Limbic association cortex	Emotion, motivation, memory.
	Wernicke's area	Speech. *Temporal lobe (dominant) lesions:* receptive aphasia.

Irene showed a mild expressive aphasia. This indicates a lesion in Broca's region. Table 7.9 shows the main types of aphasia and indicates the location of the lesions.

Table 7.9 The main types of aphasia

Type of aphasia	Site of brain damage	Compre-hension	Speech	Impaired repetition	Paraphasic errors
Broca's (*expressive*)	Motor association cortex of frontal lobe	Good	Non-fluent, agrammatical, dysarthric	Yes	Yes
Wernicke's (*receptive*)	Posterior temporal lobe	Poor	Fluent, grammatical, meaningless	Yes	Yes
Conduction	Arcuate fasciculus	Good	Fluent grammatical	Yes	Yes
Global	Substantial language area	Poor	Very little	Yes	–

The doctor then proceeded to test the integrity of the 12 cranial nerves, which are shown in Table 7.10. Complete Table 7.10. For relevant anatomy include the important foramina through which the cranial nerves emerge.

Table 7.10 Cranial nerves. Complete this table

CN	Sensory functions	Motor functions	Autonomic functions	Relevant anatomy
I (Olfactory)	Sense of smell	None	None	- - - - - - - -
II (Optic)	Vision	None	None	- - - - - - - -
III (Ophthalmic)	None	Eyeball movement		Superior orbital fissure
IV (Trochlear)	None	Eyeball movement		Superior orbital fissure
V (Trigeminal)				
VI (Abducens)	None	Eyeball movement		Superior orbital fissure
VII (Facial)				
VIII (Vestibulocochlear)				
IX (Glossopharyngeal)				
X (Vagus)				
XI (Accessory)				
XII (Hypoglossal)				

We will now follow the doctor as he examines the cranial nerves one by one. These will not necessarily be described in numerical order.

He began by enquiring about her sense of smell (CN I). She replied that there were no problems.

Which structures are responsible for olfaction?

The doctor then tested the cranial nerves involved in vision. These are CN II, III, IV and VI. He tested the integrity of CN II by testing her visual acuity and visual fields by confrontation.

How did the doctor test Irene's visual acuity and visual fields?

Figure 7.13 shows the key visual field defects.

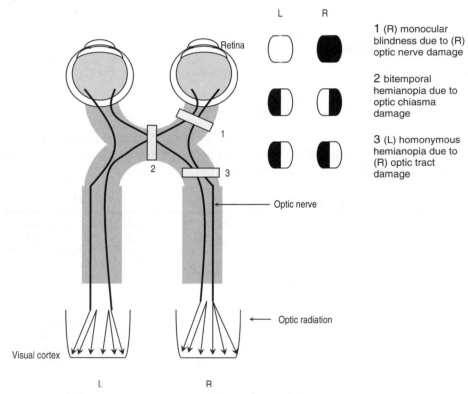

Figure 7.13   The key visual field defects

Next he tested her pupillary reaction assessing the direct and consensual reflexes. The accommodation reflex was also tested by asking her to look at a distant object and then at his index finger placed about 40 cm from her nose. Figure 7.14 shows the nerve pathways involved in the pupillary light reflex.

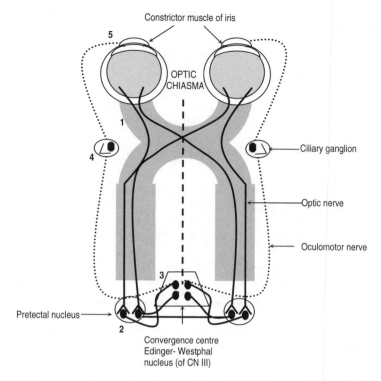

Figure 7.14 The nerve pathways involved in the pupillary light reflex. 1. Action potentials generated in the optic nerve. 2. Synapse at the pretectal nucleus. 3. Efferent pathways (not all consensual connections shown). 4. Efferent synapse in ciliary ganglion. 5. Pupillary constriction

    Describe the anatomical basis of the consensual pupillary reflex.

Her eye movements were then tested getting her to follow a moving pen. This latter test tests CN III, IV and VI.

 Can you name the muscles involved in movement of the eyeball?

You should be able to state the clinical findings observed in CN III, CN IV and CN VI lesions.

We can use the CN II, III, IV and VI examination to consider vision and the structure and function of the eye. You should be able to identify from a diagram the main structural features of the eye such as the iris, retina, sclera, etc.

Describe the location and functioning of the lacrimal apparatus

    Describe the formation of the image and the physiology of accommodation

Describe by means of diagrams, the optics of long and short sight and their correction.

Trigger box   Glaucoma

1. *Closed angle*
   Medical emergency.
   Unilateral acute closure of narrow anterior chamber angle.
   Due to pupillary dilatation, anterior uveitis, lens dislocation.
   Features: Extreme pain, blurred vision, non-reactive pupil, red eye, intraocular
   pressure (IOP) elevated.
   Treatment: Acetazolamide, pilocarpine, laser iridotomy.

2. *Open angle*
   Most common form.
   Bilateral, family history, blacks, diabetics.
   IOP elevated secondary to abnormal trabecular network. IOP rises gradually.
   Features: Initially asymptomatic, cupping of disc, progressive vision loss (peripheral
   first).
   Investigations: Tonometry, central field testing.
   Treatment: Topical beta blockers (timolol), pilocarpine, laser trabeculoplasty.

Trigger box   Retinal occlusion

Arterial/venous causes.
Features:

1. *Central artery*: sudden painless unilateral loss of vision (LOV). Poor papillary
   reactivity, cherry red spot on fovea, retinal swelling.
   Treatment: Thrombolysis, acetazolamide.

2. *Central vein*: Idiopathic, rapid, painless, retinal haemorrhages, cotton wool
   spots, fundal edema. Causes glaucoma.
   Treatment: Laser photocoagulation.

Trigger box   Macular degeneration (MD)

Leading cause of bilateral, central visual loss in elderly.
Caucasians, smokers, females, family history.
Types:

1. *Atrophic MD*: gradual vision loss.

2. *Exudative MD*: more rapid severe.

Features: Painless loss of central vision, haemorrhages in macular region.
Treatment: Laser photocoagulation may delay loss in exudative MD, verteporfin (used in the photodynamic treatment of macular degeneration with classic (no occult) subfoveal choroidal neovascularization.

What is nystagmus? Describe interpretation of abnormal nystagmus?

The doctor then tested the functioning of CN V. He tested her corneal blink reflex by touching her cornea with a wisp of cotton wool. He then tested for facial sensation testing pain and light touch. These tests were examining the sensory function of the trigeminal nerve. Irene was then asked to clench her teeth and the doctor felt her temporalis and masseter muscles. These latter tests were looking at the integrity of trigeminal motor function. Apart from an absence of pain and temperature sensation on the right side of her face the rest of her CN V examination was normal.

What does the absence of pain and temperature sensation on the right side of Irene's face indicate?
The doctor also tested Irene's jaw jerk. If it were brisker than normal what would this indicate?

The next cranial nerve tested was CN VII, the facial nerve. The doctor asked Irene to wrinkle her forehead, to shut her eyes tightly and grin.

These tests concern motor functions of CN VII. Which key sensory functions are also performed by this nerve? How are these tested?

Trigger box   Bell's palsy

Acute facial nerve palsy.
Possibly post viral.
LMN lesion.
Features: Ipsilateral weakness of facial muscles, loss of taste (anterior 2/3 of tongue), cannot close eye (pathophysiology?).
Seen in AIDS, diabetes, tumours, Lyme disease.
Treatment: Close eyelid for protection, oral steroids, aciclovir.
Most make a full recovery.

Ramsay Hunt syndrome:
Herpes zoster infection of sensory ganglion in facial canal.
LMN lesion.
Features: Facial muscle palsy, vesicles, deafness.
Treatment: Aciclovir.

Next cranial nerve VIII was tested. The cochlear and vestibular components were tested by examining hearing and balance respectively.

 By means of a diagram describe how sound is perceived.

Trigger box   Otitis media (OM)

Pathogens: *Streptococcus pneumoniae, Haemophilus influenzae, Moraxella catarrhalis*
Children more susceptible due to shorter, more horizontal Eustachian tube.
Risk factors: Viral infections, CF, Down's syndrome, immunodeficiency, cleft palate, prior OM, smoke.
Features: Fever, ear tugging, hearing loss, red bulging tympanic membrane (TM), loss of light reflex, TM can perforate.
Treatment: Analgesics. May not need antibiotics. Amoxicillin if ill with vomiting.
Complications: Meningitis, mastoiditis, hearing loss, chronic OM.

 Describe the functioning of the vestibular system.

The doctor carried out Weber and Rinne tests for conduction and sensorineural defects.

 Describe how these two tests are carried out. What is the rationale underlying these tests?

Trigger box   Vertigo

Feature: Illusion of movement of external world.
Causes: Inner ear disease (Meniere's disease, vestibular neuronitis, benign positional vertigo (BPV) or 8th nerve disease (gentamicin), brainstem tumours, infarction, multiple sclerosis (MS), migraine, cerebellar lesions.
Treatment:
Meniere's disease – betahistine, surgery.
Vestibular neuronitis – prochlorperazine.
BPV – sedatives.

The doctor next asked Irene to open her mouth. He tested for pharyngeal sensation. Here the doctor was testing CN IX.

 Which nerves are tested when the gag reflex is elicited?

He asked her to protrude her tongue. Weakness, wasting and fasciculations will be observed in damage to the hypoglossal nerve (CN XII) which is the motor nerve supplying the tongue.

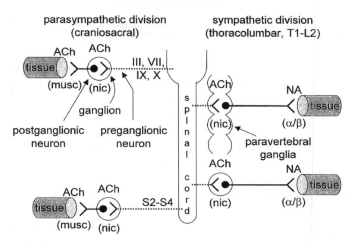

Figure 7.15 Divisions of the autonomic nervous system (nic = nicotinic, musc = muscarinic)

The doctor asked her to shrug her shoulders and rotate her head from side to side. Here he was testing the functioning of the upper trapezius and sternocleidomastoid muscles supplied by CN XI.

Let us now turn to CN X, the vagus nerve. The doctor tested the motor components of this nerve by observing palatal movements and uvular deviation.

The vagus also contains parasympathetic fibres and supplies the heart, lungs and part of the GI tract.

Parasympathetic and sympathetic nerves are constituents of the autonomic nervous system (ANS). We can consider this important branch of the nervous system next. The constituents of the ANS and their organization are depicted in Figure 7.15.

Note the pre- and postganglionic neurons and the ganglia that connect the two. Note the differences between the organization of the sympathetic and the parasympathetic nervous systems.

Preganglionic sympathetic neurons arise from thoracic and upper lumbar spinal cord (T1–L3) and form the sympathetic chain where the ganglia are located. Other sympathetic fibres synapse in nerve plexuses such as the coeliac plexus. In contrast parasympathetic preganglionic fibres arise from the brain and the sacral spinal cord.

Let us now turn to the neurotransmitters and their receptors of the autonomic nervous system. All preganglionic neurons (sympathetic and parasympathetic) are cholinergic. The acetylcholine (ACh) binds to postganglionic nicotinic receptors.

The neurotransmitters of postganglionic fibres, however, differ in sympathetic and parasympathetic systems. Sympathetic postganglionic nerves release norepinephrine (noradrenaline) and the receptors are of two types: α- and β-adrenoceptors. A small number of postganglionic sympathetic nerves also release Ach. Table 7.11 shows the distribution and functions of these receptors in different organs.

The adrenal medulla is also innervated by preganglionic sympathetic fibres which release ACh which binds to nicotinic cholinergic receptors, which stimulate

Table 7.11 The distribution and functions of adrenoceptors in different organs

Adrenoceptor	Location	Function
α_1	Smooth muscles in blood vessels supplying abdominal viscera, skin, kidneys and salivary glands; stomach and urinary bladder sphincter muscles	Vasoconstriction and sphincter closure
	Iris radial muscles	Dilatation of pupils
α_2	Smooth muscles in some blood vessels	Vasodilatation
	Pancreatic islets	Decrease insulin secretion
	Blood platelets	Aggregation
β_1	Cardiac muscle cells	Tachycardia and increased force of contraction
	Kidney juxtaglomerular cells	Secrete renin
	Salivary gland	Secrete amylase
β_2	Smooth muscles in airway walls; blood vessels supplying heart, skeletal muscle and liver; visceral organ walls	Bronchodilatation, vasodilatation and relaxation of organ walls
	Eye ciliary muscle	Relaxation
	Hepatocytes	Glycogenolysis
β_3	Brown adipose tissue	Lipolysis and thermogenesis
	Skeletal muscle	Thermogenesis

the secretion of norepinephrine (noradrenaline) and epinephrine (adrenaline), which have various α and β adrenergic effects.

Describe the 'flight or fight' reaction. What is the biological basis of this reaction?

Patients with clinical depression are treated with drugs which inhibit mono-amine oxidase (MAO). What is the rationale of this treatment strategy?

 Describe the peripheral and central effects of MAO inhibitors (MAOIs).

Postganglionic parasympathetic nerves release ACh that binds to muscarinic receptors. Table 7.12 shows the main distribution and functions of muscarinic receptors.

Autonomic transmission can be modulated by a variety of drugs.

Let us begin by considering sympathomimetics that directly or indirectly act as agonists at the postganglionic alpha and beta-receptors. Table 7.13 shows the main drug classes involved. Complete the table.

Now let us consider the key drugs that are adrenoreceptor antagonists. These are shown in Table 7.14. Complete the table.

Table 7.12 The distribution and functions of muscarinic receptors in different organs

Muscarinic receptor	Location	Function
M_1	Glands: gastric, salivary CNS: cortex, hippocampus	Gastric secretion CNS excitation
M_2	Atria, CNS	Cardiac inhibition and neuronal inhibition
M_3	Exocrine glands, smooth muscle, endothelium/blood vessels	Gastric and salivary secretion, smooth muscle contraction, vasodilatation
M_4	CNS	Enhanced locomotion
M_5	CNS: substantia nigra	Unknown

Table 7.13 Sympathomimetics. Complete the table

Drug	Receptor specificity	MOA	Indications	Toxicity
Amphetamine				
Cocaine				
Adrenaline				
Noradrenaline				
Isoprenaline				
Dopamine				
Dobutamine				
Ephedrine				
Salbutamol				
Clonidine				

MOA, mode of action.

Table 7.14 Adrenoceptor antagonists. Complete the table

Type	Receptor specificity	Indications	Toxicity
Alpha blockers			
Phenoxybenzamine			
Prazosin			
Doxasozin			
Beta blockers			
Propranolol			
Atenolol			
Timolol			

Table 7.15 shows some key drugs that are used in psychiatry. Note how the drugs increase or decrease levels of neurotransmitters that modulate the disease process.

 List the main indications and side effects of these drugs.

Table 7.15 Drugs used in psychiatry

Drug	Example	MOA
Benzodiazepines	Diazepam	↑ GABA action by ↑ Cl⁻ opening frequency
Barbiturates	Phenobarbital	↑GABA action by ↑ Cl⁻ opening duration
Neuroleptics	Haloperidol	Blocks dopamine (D2) receptors
Atypical antipsychotics	Clozapine	Blocks $5HT_2$ and dopamine receptors
Tricyclic antidepressants	Amitriptyline	Blocks 5HT and norepinephrine reuptake
SSRI	Fluoxetine	Inhibits serotonin reuptake
MAOI	Phenelzine	Non-selective MAO inhibition
Opioid analgesics	Morphine	Agonists at opioid receptors

Let us return to Irene. The doctor now began an examination of Irene's motor functions. This will enable us to consider the neurons involved in the motor pathway. We will encounter upper and lower motor neuron lesions (UMN and LMN).

Figure 7.16 shows the main motor pathways. Note the motor cortex in the precentral gyrus, the corticospinal tracts and the vestibulospinal and reticulospinal tracts. Note the upper and lower motor neurons. Table 7.16 gives features of UMN, LMN and extra-pyramidal lesions.

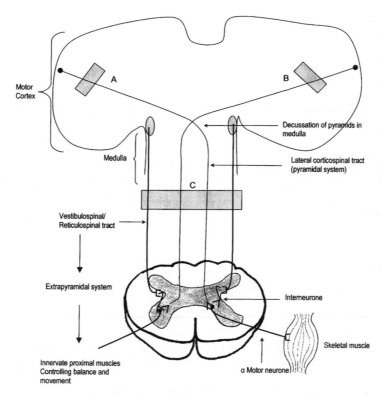

Figure 7.16 Motor pathways. Question – What are the consequences of lesions of A, B and C?

Table 7.16 Features of UMN, LMN and extrapyramidal lesions

UMN (pyramidal)	Signs on opposite side of lesion (why?). Fasciculation absent. No wasting. Spasticity &/or clonus (could have transient flaccid weakness and hyporeflexia). Weakness in arm extensors/leg flexors. Exaggerated deep tendon reflexes (DTR). Extensor plantar reflex.
Extramyramidal (basal ganglia)	Fasciculation absent. Dyskinesias. No wasting. Rigidity. Normal DTR. No integration of agonist/antagonist muscles. No weakness.
LMN	Signs same side as lesion (why?). Fasciculation present. Wasting present. Hypotonia. Weakness. Loss of DTR.

The doctor began by examining the upper limbs. He felt for muscle bulk and looked for any tenderness. He tested power at shoulders, wrists, elbows and fingers. He then proceeded to examine the biceps, triceps and brachoradialis reflexes.

If wasting and fasciculations were present in the muscles, this would indicate a LMN lesion where the pathway from the anterior horn cell is disrupted (Figure 7.16). This would however be an effect that would have taken a while to develop.

The doctor asked Irene to hold out both hands out with palms up eyes closed, observing for drifting of arms, which would have indicated an UMN lesion. If this were the case then Irene would have additionally demonstrated brisker than normal reflexes and an increase in tone. An UMN lesion could indicate damage to the nerve tracts coming from the motor area of the brain to the anterior horn cell.

Trigger box **Motor neuron disease**

Destruction of LMN, UMN and anterior horn cells in brain and spinal cord.
Imbalance in glutamate control of motor neurons implicated.
Fatal within 3 years, respiratory failure due to bulbar palsy/pneumonia.
Mainly in middle-aged men.
Findings: Fasciculation, UMN and LMN signs in three or more extremities.
Investigations: EMG, nerve conduction studies, CT/MRI.
Treatment: Supportive. Riluzole (↓ presynaptic glutamate release) may slow progression.

Irene had right-sided hemiparesis so the lesion was affecting regions of the motor cortex in the contralateral left hemisphere.

The doctor proceeded to test Irene's lower limbs in a similar manner. One of the lower limb reflexes tested was the knee jerk.

Let us now consider spinal cord reflexes. Reflex action is important in the control of muscle tone and posture. In a stretch reflex, triggered by stretching of a muscle (e.g. when the doctor tapped the quadriceps tendon) a muscle (quadriceps) contracts in response. The receptor for the stretch reflex is the muscle spindle shown in Figure 7.17(a).

This reflex is important in maintaining the resting tone of the quadriceps and will prevent the knee from buckling. The muscle spindle contains intrafusal fibres which are innervated by gamma motor neurons, which control muscle tone.

When the spindle is stretched an action potential is generated in the sensory afferent (Ia) neuron. This neuron synapses with the alpha motor neurons supplying the stretched muscle, which undergoes contraction. The sensory afferent neuron also synapses with inhibitory interneurons, which then synapse with alpha motor neurons supplying antagonistic muscles.

There are other types of reflexes, for example, withdrawal and crossed extensor reflexes. These are involved in responses to pain. Figure 7.17(b) shows the reflex arcs involved in the responses to painful stimuli.

What is the Babinski reflex? How is it tested and what is its clinical significance?

The end result of motor action is muscle contraction. Let us look at the mechanism of neuromuscular transmission and muscle contraction. A skeletal muscle contracts when an alpha motor neuron conducts an action potential which reaches a modified synapse found on the surface of the muscle fibre called the neuromuscular junction (NMJ).

The neuromuscular junction and how the action potential causes contraction are shown in Figure 7.18. The action potentials of the alpha motor neuron cause acetylcholine release, which in turn leads to a postsynaptic end plate potential (EPP), which triggers an action potential in the muscle fibre.

What are motor units?

 Define summation and tetany. Review muscle types and their different properties.

Albert had an old friend, Walter, who suffered from myasthenia gravis. Walter suffered from severe muscle fatigue due to a defective neuromuscular transmission caused by autoantibodies binding to nicotinic acetylcholine receptors. He was being treated with neostigmine which inhibited acetylcholinesterase which increases acetylcholine concentration in the NMJ.

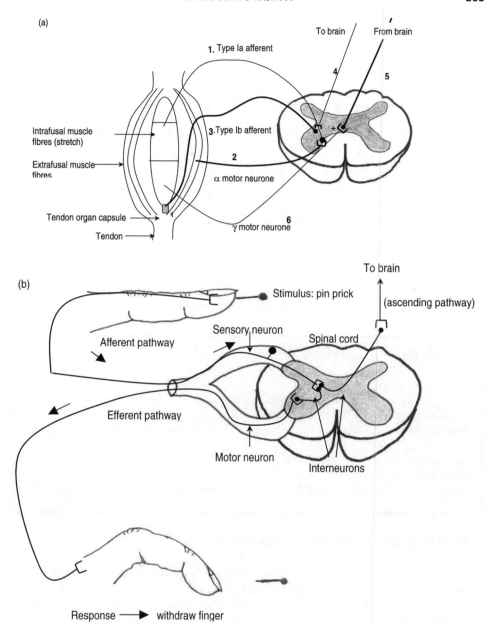

Figure 7.17 (a) Muscle spindles. Muscle stretch stimulates type 1a afferent. 2. Stimulates α motor neuron – causes contraction. 3. Type 1b afferent carries impulse from tendon organ capsule. 4. Impulse sent to CNS. 5. Impulse arrives from CNS. 6. γ motor neurone transmits impulse to extrafusal fibres. (b) Reflex arcs involved in the response to painful stimulus. Receptor activated by painful stimulus, generating action potentials in the afferent pathway. In the spinal cord, the efferent pathway causes finger to withdraw from stimulus. Interneurones carry signal on ascending pathway to the brain for pain and memory

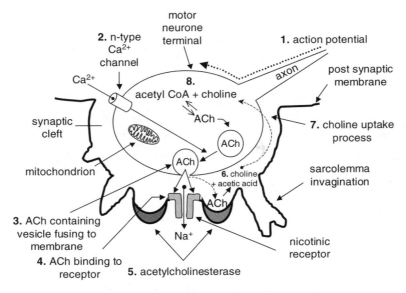

Figure 7.18   Neuromuscular junction

Trigger box   Myasthenia gravis

Female > male, Mostly in 30s.
Serum IgG against AchR in post-synaptic NMJ.
Associated with thymic hyperplasia and thymoma.
Findings: Weakness, fatigability of proximal limb, ocular and bulbar muscles, ptosis first symptom.
Anti-AchR antibodies found in 90%.
Investigations: Tensilon test, decreased evoked potentials.
Treatment: Pyridostigmine, neostigmine, thymectomy, steroids, immunosuppressives.

What is the function of acetylcholinesterase?

Let us now consider some key drugs that work on the NMJ. Some agents (e.g. hemicholinium, botulinum toxin) reduce release of acetylcholine. Others potentiate transmission by inhibiting acetylcholinesterases (pyridostigmine, neostigmine). Others block the NMJ transmission Examples are tubocurarine and suxamethonium (Table 7.17).

What are the indications of all the drugs mentioned in Table 7.17?

Albert's father worked as a farmer. In fact Albert had spent most of his childhood in the country, only having moved into the city after getting married to Irene. Albert recalled that his father had once suffered from acute organophosphate poisoning.

Table 7.17 Drugs acting on the neuromuscular junction

Specific blockade of the neuromuscular junction

A. Non-depolarizing muscular relaxants
1. Aminosteroid group, e.g. pancuronium, rocuronium and vecuronium
2. Benzylisoquinoline group, e.g. atracurium, cisatracurium, mivacurium and gallamine
Acts by competing with acetylcholine for receptor sites at the neuromuscular junction.
 Action may be reversed with anticholinesterases.

B. Depolarizing muscular relaxants
e.g. Suxamethonium
Acts by mimicking acetylcholine at the neuromuscular junction but hydrolysis is much slower.
 Cannot be reversed with anticholinesterases.

C. Botulinum toxins are specific enzymes that destroy certain of the SNARE proteins in the
 presynaptic terminals (very potent blockers).

B. Anticholinesterases
Reverse the effects of the non-depolarizing (competitive) muscle relaxant drugs.
Short-acting (e.g. edrophonium). Used in diagnosis of myasthenia gravis and suspected dual
 block due to suxamethonium.
Longer-acting (e.g. neostigmine, pyridostigmine). Used in reversing non-depolarizing
 muscular relaxants in anaesthesia and in treatment of myasthenia gravis.

*Organophosphates cause diarrhoea, urination, miosis, bronchospasm, brady-
cardia, lacrimation and sweating. Can you explain these drug effects by
considering the mechanism of action of this poison?*

*Atropine can be used to block some of these effects. What is the mechanism of
action of atropine and how does this drug reverse some symptoms of organophosphate poisoning?*

Why is benztropine used in Parkinson's disease?

Why is atropine used in bradycardia?

Why is ipratropium used in asthma and COPD?

Albert's movements are abnormal. He exhibits involuntary movements (dyskinesia),
and slowness in movement initiation (bradykinesia). These are due to a defect in his
basal ganglia. The basal ganglia are nuclei found subcortically within the forebrain. They
are involved in the control of voluntary movement via their influence on the corticospinal output but do not make direct contact with motor neurons. The outputs are via the
thalamus.

 In Albert's case a deficiency in dopamine producing neurons in the substantia nigra
and consequently reduced input is causing his movement problems.

By means of a diagram show the main inputs and outputs of the extrapyramidal
system.

Trigger box   **Huntington's disease (HD)**

AD.
Pathology: Expansion of CAG repeats in HD gene on chromosome 4 leads to mutant Huntingtin protein.
Causes loss of basal ganglia neurons.
Findings: Depletion of GABA and Ach, chorea, personality changes, dementia, death.
Symptoms begin in middle age.
No treatment.

 Chronic alcoholism can lead to the Wernicke–Korsakoff syndrome where the mamillary bodies are affected. The mamillary bodies are part of the limbic system. Describe the functions of the limbic system.

Describe the functions of the amygdala. What is Kluver–Bucy syndrome?

Let us return to Irene's neurological examination. The doctor next began testing the sensory system. The sensory pathways are shown in Figure 7.19 and are responsible for the sensation of touch, temperature, vibration, proprioception (joint position) and pain.

Note how the spinothalamic tracts cross the midline before ascending. The dorsal columns on the other hand travel on the ipsilateral side and cross over in the medulla. This crossing over has important clinical significance, for example causing contra- or ipsilateral lesions. Note the brain region in the cortex that allows conscious awareness – the somatosensory cortex located in the postcentral gyrus.

Somatosensory defects may arise because of a lesion in the peripheral nerve, in the spinal cord or within the sensory cortex.

A defective conduction in the primary sensory axons will give rise to tingling (paraesthesia) and numbness (anaesthesia). Damage to the ascending tracts is generally bilateral producing sensory loss below that level.

A stroke involving the sensory cortex will produces sensory loss on the opposite side of the body. There are usually associated motor defects.

The doctor started with the spinothalmic pathway (pain and temperature). He did this by testing the dermatomes for pain sensation by using a sharp pin. Dermatomes were shown in Chapter 6.

He then tested the dorsal (posterior) column pathway, which involves vibration sense and proprioception. Vibration was tested by placing a tuning fork on a distal intraphalengeal joint. Proprioception was tested by moving the distal phalanx and checking if the patient could correctly identify the direction of movement.

Irene had diminished pain and temperature sensation on the right side of her body, but light touch, vibration and joint position sense were normal on both sides.

 Describe the different types of sensory receptor found in the skin

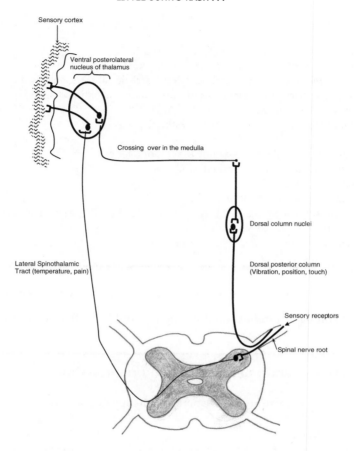

Figure 7.19 Sensory pathways

Sensory pathways also send impulses to the reticular-activating system which controls level of consciousness and sleep–wake patterns. The reticular-activating system is inhibited/damaged in coma.

Trigger box **Coma**

Central reticular formation inhibited or damaged.
Unconscious, cannot be aroused.
Glasgow Coma Scale assesses

1. eye opening.

2. verbal response.

3. motor response.

Causes of coma

CNS Disease: hypertensive encephalopathy, malaria.
Brainstem lesions: tumours, MS, trauma, Wernicke–Korsakoff.
Brainstem compression due to raised ICP: haemorrhage, abscess, encephalitis.
Metabolic: hypo/hyperglycaemia, respiratory failure, hepatic/renal failure, hypoxia, hypernatraemia, hypercalcaemia.
Toxins: drug OD, carbon monoxide, anaesthetics.
Findings
Unilateral fixed dilated pupil – coning of temporal lobe.
Bilateral fixed dilated pupil – brain death.
Papilloedema – raised ICP.
Dolls head reflex –integrity of brain stem
Investigations: CT, CSF analysis, serum glucose, U&Es, FBC, ABG, TFT, drug screen, blood culture.
Treatment: CPR, treat cause.

 Describe the sensory and motor homunculi. Explain why they look like they do.

Patients complaining of numbness and/or tingling could be suffering from a vitamin B_{12} deficiency.

Trigger box   **Vitamin deficiencies and neuropathy**

NB. In malnutrition, there are usually multiple vitamin deficiencies.

1. *Thiamine* (B_1)
   Features: Wernicke–Korsakoff, beri-beri (polyneuropathy, encephalopathy, cardiac failure).
   Treatment: Thiamine.

2. *Pyridoxine* (B_6)
   Features: Sensory neuropathy.
   Causes: Isoniazid therapy.
   Treatment: B_6.

3. *Vitamin B_{12}*
   Features: Subacute combined degeneration of the cord (distal sensory loss, absent ankle jerks, brisk knee jerk, extensor plantar.
   Treatment: B_{12} reverses peripheral nerve damage.

4. *Folate*
   Features: Neural tube defects.
   Treatment: Folate before conception and first 12 weeks of pregnancy.

Next, the doctor examined the saddle region for sensation and also tested the anal reflex.

What lesions cause foot drop?

Coordination was then tested with a heel–shin, nose–finger test. The doctor also carried out the Romberg test to check Irene's cerebellar function.

 Describe the Romberg test.

The cerebellum plays a major role in the control of motor function. Cerebellar contacts are required for balance and smooth coordinated movements. Cerebellar lesions are indicated by loss of balance and unsteady gait. Patients cannot perform rapid alternating movements. In Irene's case there were no signs of cerebellar dysfunction.

Irene underwent a head MRI, which revealed the location of the insult.

Where is the lesion most likely to be?

She was admitted and placed under regular observation, e.g. hourly BP checks. She was treated with diuretics to control her BP. She was mobilized after her first day but found walking difficult. Her speech improved. However, 2 days later Irene suffered a small seizure.

Trigger box   Epilepsy

Epilepsy = tendency to have seizures.
2% of UK population.
75% idiopathic.
30% have first degree relative.
Causes: head injury, surgery, infarction, tumours, encephalitis, chronic meningitis, drug OD, alcohol withdrawal, metabolic disturbances.
Status epilepticus = 2 or more seizures without regaining of consciousness.
Investigations: EEG, CT/MRI.
Types

1. *Generalized*
   Tonic–clonic (grand mal): seconds to minutes, tongue-biting, incontinence, postictal.
   Absence (petit mal): seconds; 3 Hz spike and wave.
   Myoclonic: involuntary muscle jerks.
   Treatment: Phenobarbital, phenytoin, carbamazepine, sodium valproate, lamotrigine.
   Absence: ethosuximide.

2. *Partial*
   Simple: consciousness preserved, e.g. Jacksonian, Todd's paralysis.
   Complex: LOC, e.g. temporal lobe seizures, olfactory/visual hallucinations, jamais-vu, déjà-vu
   Treatment: Carbamazepine, phenytoin, valproate.

What about Albert? Albert's Parkinsonism responded (initially at least) to co-careldopa. Within a few weeks he and the family noticed a marked improvement in his movements. His facial features were more expressive and his handwriting improved. His tremor too improved significantly.

8

The reproductive system

Learning strategy

In this chapter we will consider the essential, 'must know' facts and concepts of the reproductive system. Our main strategy would involve an exploration of these key principles by following a pregnancy.

A physical examination carried out as part of an investigation for infertility will introduce you to the anatomical features of the reproductive system. Hormonal tests will introduce gametogenesis. A scenario involving erectile dysfunction will lead to the mechanics of sexual intercourse. Following a pregnancy from conception to birth will allow consideration of fertilization, implantation and key fetal developmental stages.

We will consider maternal physiology and the stages of labour, culminating in the birth. Breast-feeding and lactation will be discussed. Finally, a short scenario will lead to a discussion of the menopause.

Throughout, we will also consider the pathophysiological mechanisms of several key disease states involving the reproductive system which will, in addition to high-lighting the key pathophysiological principles, further reinforce basic principles of anatomy, physiology and pharmacology relevant to the reproductive system.

Try to answer the questions and try to complete the Learning Tasks.

Debbie's changes . . .

Debbie was 11 years of age when she noticed the beginning of breast growth. Around this time she was also growing fast in both her height and weight. She also noticed the first signs of pubic hair: these first hairs started out fine and straight, rather than curly. Over

Integrated Medical Sciences by Shantha Perera, Stephen Anderson, Ho Leung and Rousseau Gama
© 2007 John Wiley & Sons, Ltd ISBN: 978470016589 (HB) 978470016596 (PB)

the next months the breast growth continued and her pubic hair became coarser and somewhat darker. Around 7 months later she noticed that the pubic hair growth had taken on an inverted triangular shape. She also found that hair was starting to grow under her armpits. She experienced her first period 6 months later. 'So is it going to happen at the same time next month?' she asked Mary

'Sort of, but you won't get a regular cycle for awhile yet' Mary replied.

What are the Tanner Stages

Debbie's puberty sets the stage for our discussion of the reproductive system. We will begin by considering the development of the male and female reproductive systems. Both systems begin developing during fetal life. The key developmental stages are shown in Figure 8.1.

Note that the mesonephric (Wolffian) ducts form the male structures while the paramesonephric (Mullerian) ducts form the female structures.

The Y chromosome causes the primitive gonads to become testes. Testosterone produced by the testes then causes the development of the male sex organs. The important antimullerian hormone secreted by the testes inhibit the formation of the female reproductive organs by the mullerian duct. When the Y chromosome is absent, the primitive gonads develop into ovaries and other female organs are also formed.

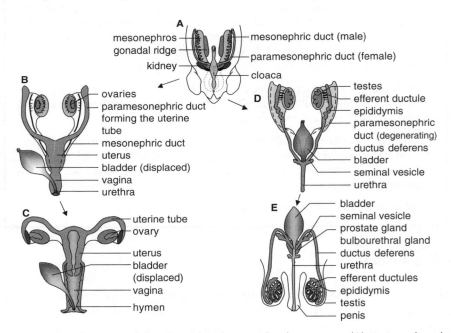

Figure 8.1 Development of female and male reproductive organs. (A) 5–6 week embryo, (B) 8–9 week female fetus, (C) female at birth, (D) 7–8 week male fetus, (E) male at birth. Adapted from Tortora and Grabowski (2003), Principles of Anatomy and Physiology, 10th edition, John Wiley & Sons

Table 8.1 Genital homologues

Male	Female
Scrotum	Labia majora
	Labia minora
	Clitoris
Prostate gland	
Cowper's gland	Bartholin's gland
Corpus spongiosus	Vestibular bulbs

Table 8.1 shows male and female structures derived from similar origins. Complete the table.

Table 8.2 shows the secondary sexual characteristics and the main changes taking place during puberty.

In both males and females gonadotrophin releasing hormone (GnRH) produced by the hypothalamus stimulates the anterior pituitary to release the gonadotrophins, follicle-stimulating hormone (FSH) and luteinizing hormone (LH). FSH and LH in turn cause development of the gonads and spermatogenesis and oogenesis, which we shall consider later. The subsequent increase in testosterone and oestrogens by the developing gonads are responsible for the appearance of the secondary sexual characteristics of males and females respectively.

 Describe the main types of congenital penile abnormalities.

Table 8.2 Secondary sexual characteristics and the main changes taking place during puberty

Characteristic	Female change	Male change
Hair	Development of pubic, axillary and some body hair	Development of pubic, axillary, facial, body and in some cases chest hair
Voice	Feminization of voice	Deepening due to larynx enlargement
Sex hormones	Rising levels of oestrogen	Increasing levels of testosterone
Growth	Widening and lightening (feminization) of the pelvis. Increased deposit of subcutaneous fat	Increased bone growth and density. Increased skeletal muscle development
Genitalia	Growth and maturation of internal and external genitalia	Enlargement of testes and scrotum. Growth of penis
Breast	Growth of breasts	

Debbie wants a baby...

It is 10 years since Debbie's puberty and things have certainly moved on for her and Max who have been together for just over 2 years now. They appear to have a stable relationship. Debbie has got steady work as a hairdresser and Max has found work in a music shop.

But all was not well. Debbie wanted a baby. But in spite of trying Debbie couldn't get pregnant, which is what brought her to Dr Smith. . .

Dr Smith began by taking a history. He enquired about her menstrual cycles. She commented that her last menstrual period was 3 weeks ago. Her cycles have never really been regular and she was having heavy periods, which went on for about 12 days.

What are the main causes of heavy/irregular periods?

They were having sex regularly, three to four times a week, she added ruefully, but without success. She also commented about her rapid weight gain and facial hair and expressed her concerns that Max may be 'going off' her.

Dr Smith reviewed her past notes. Debbie had had infrequent periods since 13. She had been prescribed the combined oral contraceptive pill to make her periods more regular but she had stopped the pill because of weight gain.

Trigger box   Contraceptive pills

1. *Oral progestogen-only contraceptives (mini-pill)*
   Must use continuously every day at the same time.
   Mode of action: Making cervical mucus unfavourable to sperm, reducing tubal motility. Also can inhibit ovulation.
   Side effects: PV spotting. Increase risk of ectopic pregnancy.

2. *Combined hormonal contraceptives*

Mode of action

1. suppression of gonadotrophins by oestrogen.

2. progestogen effects as in minipill.
   Side effects: Nausea, vomiting, headaches, breast tenderness, fluid retention, thrombosis, changes in libido, depression, cloasma, hypertension, impairment of liver function, hepatic tumour.

How does mifepristone work?
What is in the 'morning after pill'? What is its MOA?

 Find out about other methods of contraception.

Debbie *had* become pregnant when she was 17. Dr Smith noted the termination, which had taken place after 12 weeks. After that she had had a coil fitted for a short period but had asked it to be removed due to dysmenorrhoea. She had then been prescribed the combined pill again.
Endometriosis is a common cause of dysmenorrhoea.

Trigger box Endrometriosis

Endometrial tissue outside uterus (e.g. ovaries).

Most common cause of dysmenhorrhoea.

Possible causes: Retrograde menstruation, blood/lymph spread.

Risk factors: Family history, nulliparity, infertility.

Features: Premenstrual and pelvic pain, dyschezia, dyspareunia, infertility, bleeding, nodular uterosacral ligament, fixed retroverted uterus, adnexal masses.

Investigations: Laparoscopy – chocolate cysts, raspberry lesions.

Treatment: Combined OCP, GnRH analogues, hormone replacement treatment (HRT), surgery (laser vaporization, TAH-BSO (total abdominal hysterectomy/bilateral salphingo-oophorectomy).

Dr Smith noted that some 6 months after the termination Debbie had presented with vaginal discharge and painful intercourse. Her abdominal examination had revealed bilateral lower abdominal pain but without guarding or rebound. She had also been afebrile. Her gynaecological examination had revealed a normal vulva and perineum but there was a yellowish vaginal discharge. Digital vaginal examination had revealed cervical motion tenderness and some bilateral adnexal tenderness. He had, however, not detected any masses. The endocervix had shown contact bleeding and he had taken samples for bacterial culture and sensitivity and for *Chlamydia* antigens. The swab had revealed *Chlamydia*. Debbie was treated with doxycycline and had made a full recovery. Debbie and Max had subsequently attended the local genitourinary medicine clinic and both were found to be clear of other STDs.

Trigger box Gonorrhoea

Gram-negative intracellular diplococcus *Neisseria gonorrhoeae*.

Infects epithelium of urinogenital tract, pharynx, rectum, conjunctivae.

Incubation period 7 days.

80–90% women contract disease after single encounter compared to 20–25 % men.

Findings: Yellow–green discharge, adnexal pain, swollen Bartholin's abscess, dysuria, urethral meatus oedema, prostatitis, rash, arthritis.

Investigations: Gram stain discharge, endocervical swab- culture on Thayer–Martin agar.

Treatment: Ceftriaxone i.m., ciprofloxacin.

Complications: Infertility, tuboovarian abscess (TOA).

Trigger box   Chlamydial infections

Most common bacterial STD.

C. trachomatis.

Infect urinogenital tract, anus, eye, can coexist with gonorrhoea.

Incubation period = 21 days.

Common cause of non-gonococcal urethritis (NGU) in men.

Findings: Often asymptomatic. Urethritis, mucopurulent cervicitis, salpingitis, abdominal pain, fever, mucopurulent cervical discharge, penile discharge (clear), testicular tenderness, conjunctivitis and pneumonia in newborn.

Investigations: Urine PCR.

Treatment: Doxycycline or azithromycin. Erythromycin if pregnant.

Complications: Chronic infection, Reiter's syndrome, Fitz Hugh Curtis syndrome, pelvic inflammatory disease (PID), infertility, epididymitis.

What are the other infections caused by *Chlamydia*?

Trigger box   Syphilis

Treponema pallidum.

Transmission: sexual intercourse, transplacental.

Stages:

Primary: (10–90 days); chancre, heals in 3–9 weeks.

Secondary: (4–10 weeks after chancre); fever, headache, lymphadenopathy, maculopapular rash soles/palm, condylomata lata, arthalgias, snail track ulcers.

Lesions heal in 2–6 weeks.

Tertiary: (1–20 years) granulamatous gummas in skin, bone, liver, testes. Tabes dorsalis, Argyll Robertson pupil, aortitis, aortic aneurysms, aortic regurgitation.

Investigations: Dark field microscopy, VDRL/RPR, FTA-ABS/MHA-TP.

Treatment: Procaine benzylpenicillin i.m. (beware of Jarisch–Herxheimer reaction).

Tetracycline/doxycycline (penicillin resistant).

Intravenous penicillin for neurosyphilis.

VDRL/RPR = venereal disease research laboratory/rapid plasma reagin; FTA-ABS = fluorescent treponemal antibody-absorbed; MHA-TP = microhaemaggluntination assay *Treponema pallidum.*

Dr Smith also noted that Debbie's latest cervical PAP smear had been normal.

Trigger box   Cervical cancer

Third most common gynaecological malignancy.

Mainly squamous cell carcinoma.

Precursor – cervical dysplasia.

Risk factors: Early sex; multiple partners, HIV, STDs, smoking, HPV (16, 18, 31).

Features: Can be asymptomatic, dysmenorrhagia, postcoital bleeding, discharge, pelvic pain, cervical changes.

Investigations: Colposcopy, endocervical curettage.

Prognosis: 65% 5 year survival.

Types

Invasive: Treat by radial hysterectomy, lymph node removal, radiation, chemotherapy.

Cervical intraepithelial neoplasia (CIN)

CIN I (atypical cells in lower 1/3) mild dysplasia – can regress spontaneously. Observe.

CIN II (atypical cells in lower 2/3) moderate. Treat as CIN III.

CIN III (atypical cells in full thickness) severe: treat by cryosurgery, loop electrocautery excision, cold knife conization.

Prevention: HPV vaccine, screening: PAP smear.

Trigger box   Vaginitis

Change in normal acidic vaginal pH predisposes to infection.

Measure vaginal pH, wet prep, Gram stain.

Pathogens

1. Bacterial vaginosis

   Gardnerella vaginalis, polymicrobial.

   Features: Greyish discharge; fishy stale odour, vulval irritation.

   Clue cells, vaginal pH >4.5.

   Investigations: Whiff test.

   Treatment: Metronidazole.

   Complication: PID.

2. *Trichomonas vaginalis*

   STD.

   Features: Greenish, frothy discharge; strawberry petechiae in cervix.

   pH > 4.5.

   Treatment: Metronidazole.

3. *Candida*

   Features: Thick white discharge, pruritis, erythematous.

   Pseudohyphae.

   Treatment: Miconazole, fluconazole.

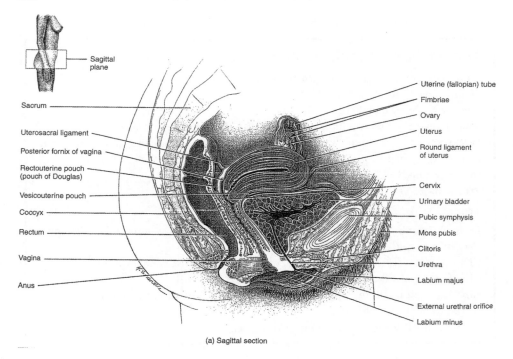

(a) Sagittal section

Figure 8.2 Female Reproductive System. Adapted from Tortora and Grabowski (2003), Principles of Anatomy and Physiology, 10th Edition, John Wiley and Sons Inc. New York

Dr Smith began his physical examination. Debbie was obese at 87 kg, and her BMI was 33 kg/m^2. He noted a little facial hair. Her breasts were normal. Vaginal examination indicated a normal cervix and a normal anteverted uterus. There were no adnexal masses.

?   *Is Debbie's BMI within the normal range?*

Debbie's physical examination leads us to a consideration of the main anatomical features of the female reproductive system. The main structures are shown in Figure 8.2.

?   *Can you relate the structure of the uterus to its function?*

Trigger box   Fibroids

Very common: benign smooth muscle tumour, hormonally responsive.

Increases in size during pregnancy.

Leiomyosarcoma transformation very rare (0.5%).

Black female, age >35.

Features: Asymptomatic, abnormal uterine bleeding, dysmenorrhoea, lumpy uterus on examination.

Investigation: Ultrasound scan.

Treatment: Hysteroscopic resection, embolization, myomectomy, hysterectomy if severe, tranexamic acid, GnRH agonists, progesterone, danazol.

'We need to do more tests to find out why you are not getting pregnant' Dr Smith told Debbie after the physical examination. 'We need to check Max as well. Could you ask him to drop in and see me?'...

Max was less than enthusiastic but agreed to visit the surgery. He arrived for his appointment a week later.

Dr Smith glanced through Max's file, noting his rather colourful history peppered with numerous accidents and misadventures with non-prescription drugs. 'I have stopped all that', Max declared. 'I've been clean for nearly 3 years'. Dr Smith noted that there was no recorded history of a prior STD.

Max's physical examination was unremarkable and revealed normal external genitalia.

'Do you wear tight pants? Take very hot baths?' Dr Smith asked. Max gave him a bemused look and shook his head. 'Have you had mumps in the past?' Dr Smith asked. Max shrugged his shoulders, which Dr Smith took to indicate a no. Dr Smith wrote out a semen analysis request form and told him that he would refer Debbie to the fertility clinic if his sperm count was normal.

What was the significance of Dr Smith's questions?

We can now look at the male reproductive system. Figure 8.3 shows the main anatomical structures. Spermatogenesis takes place in the seminiferous tubules whilst testosterone is produced by interstitial Leydig cells. Fetal testosterone causes the descent of the testes through the inguinal canal; hence at birth they lie inside the scrotum.

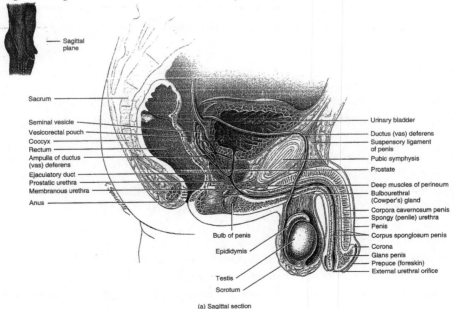

(a) Sagittal section

Figure 8.3 Male Reproduction System. Adapted from Tortora and Grabowski (2003), Principles of Anatomy and Physiology, 10th Edition, John Wiley and Sons Inc. New York

What is the significance of the testes descending into the scrotum?
What are the consequences of undescended testes?

Now that we have considered the anatomical features of the male and female reproductive systems, we can turn to their functions.

Debbie and Max visit the fertility clinic

Debbie and Max saw Dr Dobbs the consultant at the fertility clinic at Hope Hospital. Dr Dobbs began by reviewing the blood test results sent to him by Dr Smith.

Debbie's hormonal profile indicated normal serum testosterone but decreased sex hormone binding protein (SHBG) and a high LH/FSH ratio. The prolactin and thyroid-stimulating hormone (TSH) levels were normal. He ordered an ultrasound scan and laparoscopy.

What do you think is the significance of the high FSH/LH ratio?
Why were prolactin levels and thyroid function assessed?

The abdominal ultrasound scan showed enlarged ovaries and several small peripheral cysts with increased stroma consistent with polycystic ovaries (PCOS). Laparoscopy confirmed polycystic ovaries and a normal sized uterus. There were some pelvic adhesions suggestive of previous pelvic infection. Dye insufflation indicated a slow delayed spill on the right fallopian tube side but no spill from the left fallopian tube.

Trigger box   Polycystic ovarian syndrome

Age 15–30.

Features:

Androgenism: Hirsutism and acne.

Menstrual disturbance: Amenorrhoea, oligomenorrhoea and dysfunctional uterine bleeding, infertility, anovulation.

Central obesity.

Hypertension, acanthosis nigrans.

Insulin resistance, diabetes, increased endometrial cancer risk

Findings: Excess LH, Increased ovarian and adrenal androgens: testosterone, androstenedione and dehydroepiandrostenedione (DHEA) and DHEA sulphate (DHEAS). Low SHBG, LH/FSH > 3.

Physical exam: Enlarged cystic ovaries.

Investigations: Ultrasound shows enlarged ovaries, thickened capsule, 10 or more 3–5 mm peripheral cysts and a hyperechogenic stroma.

Treatment: Weight reduction, clomiphene (infertility) metformin, OCP, cyproterone acetate, finasteride (hirsutism).

Debbie's previous *Chlamydia* infection could have led to pelvic inflammatory disease, which is an important cause of infertility.

Trigger box   Pelvic inflammatory disease (PID)

A spectrum of infections of the female genital tract.

Includes endometritis, salpingitis, tubo-ovarian abscess, and peritonitis.

PID is caused by organisms such as *Chlamydia trachomatis* and *Neisseria gonorrhoeae* ascending to the upper female genital tract from the vagina and cervix.

Features: Lower abdominal tenderness on palpation, adnexal tenderness and cervical motion tenderness. Fever, abnormal cervical or vaginal discharge may be present.

Investigations: ESR and CRP (elevated), test for cervical infection with *N. gonorrhoeae* and *C. trachomatis*.

Complications: Chronic pelvic pain is common in about 18% after a single episode. Tubal occlusion.

Infertility occurs at a rate of 12–50%, increasing with each episode of PID.

Ectopic pregnancy rates are 12–15% higher.

Treatment: ofloxacin, metronidazole, ceftriaxone, doxycycline.

Dr Dobbs, the consultant discussed the findings with Debbie. He mentioned that the difficulty in achieving a pregnancy could be due to a combination of factors, namely the pelvic adhesions and PCOS.

Debbie's investigations involved analysis of FSH and LH levels. We can now consider the functions of these key hormones. They are involved in the process of oogenesis, which is shown in Figure 8.4. The ovarian and uterine cycles are depicted in Figure 8.5. Note the proliferative and secretory phases. Figure 8.5 also shows the hormonal changes during these cycles. The functions and feedback controls of these key hormones are further detailed in Figure 8.6. Study these figures and try to answer the questions given below.

Which factor causes the LH surge, which stimulates ovulation?
Which factors then cause a subsequent decline in LH and FSH?

Describe the endocrine functions of the corpus luteum.

Functions of oestrogens and progesterome are shown in Table 8.3.

Let us consider the uterine cycle. Note how the endometrium thins out during menstruation. Following this, increasing oestrogen levels stimulate endometrial hyperplasia. After ovulation progesterone causes development of the glands within the endometrium. In this secretory phase the glands also secrete glycogen, these

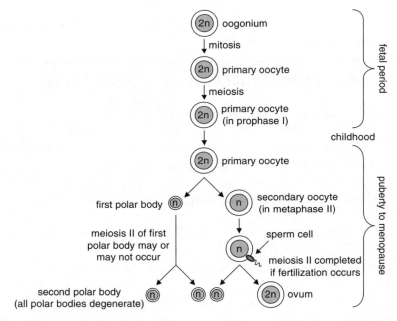

Figure 8.4   Oogenesis. 2n = diploid number (46), n = haploid number (23). Adapted from Tortora and Grabowski (2003), Principles of Anatomy and Physiology, 10th edition, John Wiley & Sons

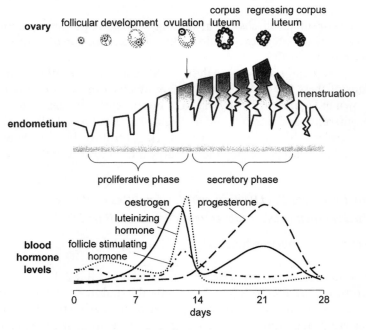

Figure 8.5   Ovarian and uterine cycles. Adapted from McGeown (1999) Physiology, Churchill Livingstone

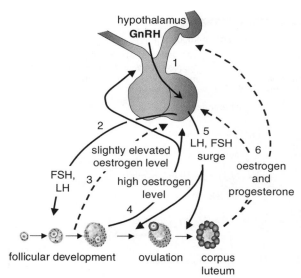

1. GnRH stimulates release of LH and FSH.
2. FSH and LH stimulates follicular development.
3. oestrogen negatively feeds back on FSH, LH and GnRH.
4. high oestrogen levels positively feeds back on LH secretion.
5. LH (mainly) surge causes ovulation.
6. Increasing oestrogen and progesterone negatively feed back on LH and FSH secretion.

Figure 8.6 Hormonal control of female reproductive cycle. Solid lines = stimulation, dashed lines = inhibition. Adapted from Tortora and Grabowski (2003), Principles of Anatomy and Physiology, 10th edition, John Wiley & Sons

changes preparing the uterus for possible implantation. If pregnancy does not occur the rapid decline in oestrogen and progesterone following atresia of the corpus luteum cause destruction of the endometrium, which is shed during the next menstrual cycle.

Table 8.3 Functions of oestrogens and progesterone

Oestrogen
    Development of genitalia & breast
    Follicular growth
    Proliferation of endometrium
    Increased myometrial excitability
    Fat distribution (female)
    LH surge, feedback inhibition of FSH

Progesterone
    Inhibition of LH, FSH
    Decreased myometrial excitability
    Spiral artery development
    Maintenance of pregnancy
    Breast development
    Production of sperm inhibiting cervical mucus
    Relaxation of uterine smooth muscle
    Stimulation of endometrial secretions

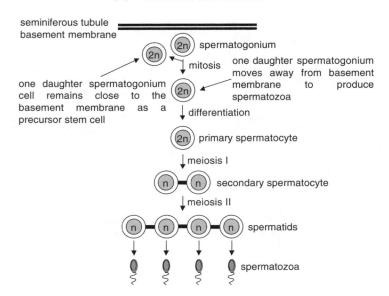

Figure 8.7   Spermatogenesis. 2n = diploid number (46), n = haploid number (23). Adapted from Tortora and Grabowski (2003), Principles of Anatomy and Physiology, 10th edition, John Wiley & Sons

Dr Dobbs explained that Max's sperm count had been satisfactory with 85 per cent showing normal morphology and 80 per cent, good, progressive motility.

What is a normal sperm count? What are the functions of the various constituents of semen?

Max's semen analysis allows us to consider spermatogenesis, which is shown in Fig 8.7. Hormonal control of spermatogenesis is shown in Figure 8.8.

Note the many similarities to the processes in the female reproductive system and the feedback cycles. Testosterone functions are shown in Table 8.4.

Dr Dobbs advised Debbie and Max that female and male factors can cause infertility but in their case, the infertility was most likely caused by female factors.

Trigger Box   Infertility

Cannot conceive after 1 year.

Male factors (30–40%); female factors (60–70%).

Other factors: Tubal factors (from PID or endometriosis), cervical factors, ovulatory factors (PCOS, hypothalamic hypogonadism, hyperprolactinaemia).

Investigations: Semen analysis, serum FSH/LH/TSH/prolactin, hysterosalpingography, luteal phase progesterone.

The most common female infertility factor is an ovulation disorder (see Table 8.5).

Treatment: See Table 8.6.

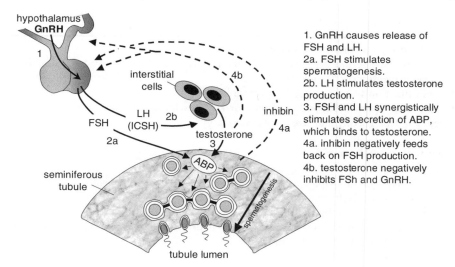

1. GnRH causes release of FSH and LH.
2a. FSH stimulates spermatogenesis.
2b. LH stimulates testosterone production.
3. FSH and LH synergistically stimulates secretion of ABP, which binds to testosterone.
4a. inhibin negatively feeds back on FSH production.
4b. testosterone negatively inhibits FSh and GnRH.

Figure 8.8 Hormonal control of spermatogenesis. ABP = androgen binding protein. Solid lines = stimulation, dashed lines = inhibition. Adapted from Tortora and Grabowski (2003), Principles of Anatomy and Physiology, 10th edition, John Wiley & Sons

He advised them on the options available and the possibility of IVF, which he mentioned could involve involved intracytoplasmic sperm injection. The couple wanted to give IVF a try. Table 8.5 shows how infertility is assessed.

Table 8.6 shows some important drugs used in the treatment of infertility. Note that these can cause ovarian hyperstimulation and multiple gestation.

Table 8.4 Functions of testosterone

Effects	Principal actions
Pre-parturition	Masculinization of external genitalia and reproductive tract. Promotion of testicle descent into the scrotum.
Sex-specific tissues	Promotion of growth and maturation of the reproductive system at puberty. Spermatogenesis. Maintains adult reproductive tract.
Reproduction	Development of sex drive. Regulation of gonadotropin hormone secretion.
Secondary sexual characteristics	Promotion of muscle growth. Induction of male pattern hair growth. Thickening of vocal folds and deepending of voice.
Non-reproductive	Protein anabolism. Promotion of bone growth and eventual epiphyseal plate closure. Increased aggression.

Table 8.5   Assessment of infertility

Women with regular menstrual cycle
Mid-luteal phase serum progesterone (>30 nmol/L) to confirm ovulation (7 days before
  onset of menses; day 21 for 28 day cycle)
Thyroid function tests: primary hypothyroidism
Tubal patency tests: hysterosalpingogram or hysterosalpingo-contrast-ultrasonography
Diagnostic laparoscopy and dye: pelvic pathology

Women with oligo/amenorrhoea
(Pregnancy test)
FSH, LH: hypogonadotrophic and hypergonadotrophic hypogonadism
Prolactin: hyperprolactinaemia
Thyroid function: hypothyroidism
Suspected hyperandrogenism: testosterone, 17-hydroxyprogesterone: PCOS, congenital
  adrenal hyperplasia, androgen tumours

Men
Seminal fluid analysis
Serum LH, FSH and testosterone if repeated azoospermia is present

Table 8.6   Treatment of infertility

Ovulation induction	Anti-oestrogens: Clomiphene Gonadotrophins: FSH and LH or HCG Pulsatile gonadotropin releasing hormone: Metformin for PCOS Dopamine agonists for hyperprolactinaemia Laparoscopic ovarian drilling: Failure of medical treatment in PCOS
Surgical treatment	Tubal surgery Tubal disease Laparoscopic surgery: endometriosis Surgery for fibroids Surgical correction of epididymal blockage
Assisted conception	Intra-uterine insemination (IUI) Donor insemination (DI) *In vitro* fertilization (IVF) Intracytoplasmic sperm injection (ICSI) Oocyte donation. Embryo donation. Gamete intrafallopian transfer (GIFT)

Do you understand the rationale underlying all these different strategies?

So far we have considered the anatomy of the male and female reproductive systems, the processes of gametogenesis and the ovarian and uterine cycles. However, for fertilization to take place a sperm must meet an ovum. In the case of Max and Debbie this involved an *in vitro* process. However, in the normal state of affairs, sexual intercourse is the mechanism that allows fertilization to occur. Sexual intercourse involves the important processes of erection and ejaculation and we can look at these by considering John's problem.

John has a new embarrassing problem ...

John was not a happy man. His sex life, which wasn't great at the best of times, had quite literally taken a dip. Lately he was having erection problems. He could achieve an erection but it did not last long enough to achieve penetration. He went to see Dr Smith.

Dr Smith was sympathetic and explained that the problem could be due to his underlying medical condition and/or his medication.

 Considering John's medical history, what is the likely mechanism causing John's erectile dysfunction?
What are the main causes of erectile dysfunction.? How does sildenafil work?

John's unfortunate difficulties lead us to consider the mechanics of sexual intercourse. Erection is caused by vascular engorgement, which in turn is caused by psychological erotic stimuli and tactile stimulation of mechanoreceptors on the glans penis. The ensuing spinal reflex causes activation of parasympathetic nerves and inhibition of sympathetic nerves.

During ejaculation a sympathetic nerve reflex causes contraction of epididymal and vas deferens smooth muscle, which results in the propulsion of semen. Rhythmical contraction of skeletal muscle at the base of the penis causes discharge.

Debbie is pregnant!

The IVF worked after three agonizing attempts. There had been a lot of delays, stresses, disappointments, inconveniences of attending clinics for ultrasound scans and operations, and the pain from injections. But Debbie forgot all this and got really excited when she missed her period by a week. A pregnancy test turned out positive.

 describe the basis of the pregnancy test.

Trigger box   **Gestational trophoblastic disease**

Hydatiform mole (benign), choriocarcinoma (malignant).

Complete moles – sperm fertilizing empty ovum and undergoing mitosis, 46XX (most), paternally derived.

Incomplete moles – two sperm fertilizing normal ovum; 69XXY (80%) or 69XXX (20%). Has fetal tissue.

Risk factors: age (<20 or > 40), folate/beta carotine deficiency, blood group incompatibilities.

Can progress to invasive moles (12%) and choriocarcinoma (3%).

Features: Pre-eclampsia, uterine bleeding (1st trimester), hyperemesis gravidum.

Can progress to lung or CNS metastases, pulmonary emboli.

Findings: Uterine size > gestational age, No fetal heartbeat, greatly elevated β-HCG, snowstorm on US.

Treatment: ERPOC (evacuation of retained product of conception), chemotherapy, radiotherapy, hysterectomy.

Debbie cried when the radiographer told her that there was a possible gestational sac inside the uterus. At 8 weeks' gestation when they attended the fertility clinic the last time for a scan, Debbie and Max were relieved to learn that the fetal heartbeat was finally detectable and there was only one fetus. Debbie went to see Dr Smith with the good news and a photograph of her latest ultrasound scan. She had a problem though, morning sickness. . .

?   *What could be causing Debbie's morning sickness?*

Hyperemesis gravidum is an intractable form of morning sickness.

Trigger box   **Hyperemesis gravidum**

Severe nausea & vomiting persisting beyond 14–16 weeks.

Can cause dehydration, hypokalaemic–hypochloraemic metabolic alkalosis, hyponatraemia.

More common in nulliparas, molar pregnancies.

Treatment: Antiemetics, small meals; may require i.v. fluids.

In the normal state of affairs, of the 300 million sperm released during a normal ejaculation less than 5per cent enter the uterus. The mucus plug covering the cervical canal thins out around ovulation allowing sperm to swim through it. Uterine contractions cause sperm to proceed and some enter the fallopian tubes. Fertilization normally occurs in the lateral 1/3 of the fallopian tube. Sometimes, however, implantation can occur outside the uterus!

> ### *Trigger box* Ectopic pregnancy
>
> Implantation outside uterus.
>
> Ampulla of oviduct most common site (95%).
>
> **Risk factors**: PID, prior ectopic pregnancy, surgery, DES exposure, IUD.
>
> **Features:** Amenorrhoea, vaginal bleeding, lower abdominal pain, tender pelvic/adnexal mass, infertility, rupture –shock.
>
> **Investigations:** Measure serial β-HCG, transabdominal/transvaginal US, laparoscopy/laparatomy.
>
> **Treatment:** Methotrexate, surgery.

For fertilization to occur the spermatozoan must penetrate the corona radiata and zona pellucida that suround the ovum.

describe the process of capacitation.

describe the acrosomal reaction.

Following fertilization, the zygote which becomes a morula reaches the uterus. This develops into a blastocyst which consists of an outer tropoblast cell layer a fluid filled blastocoele and an inner cell mass. The syncytiotrophoblast secretes enzymes that allow the blastocyst to digest endometrial tissue in order to implant (Figure 8.9). The cells of

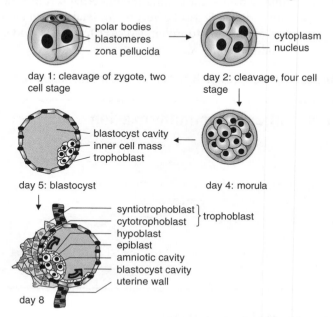

Figure 8.9 Formation of the blastocyst. Adapted from Tortora and Grabowski (2003), Principles of Anatomy and Physiology, 10th edition, John Wiley & Sons

Table 8.7 Common prenatal tests carried out in pregnancy

Ultrasonography (dating scan at 12 weeks; anomaly scan at 20 weeks)
Amniocentesis if indicated
Chorionic villus sampling if indicated
Fetal blood cells in maternal blood
Maternal serum alpha-fetoprotein
Maternal serum β-HCG
Maternal serum oestriol

HCG, human chorionic gonadotrophin.

the inner cell mass differentiate into the hypoblast and epiblast, which together form the bilaminar embryonic disc.

After around 10 days following fertilization the blastocyst implants into the endometrium.

Dr Smith congratulated Debbie and referred her to the ante-natal clinic, which she attended the following week. She was given a routine checkup, which did not reveal anything unusual, except a BP of 139/84. Theresa, the midwife noted that the uterus was not palpable per abdomen and was consistent with the last menstrual period (LMP) date. A urine dipstick found a trace of protein. Bloods were drawn for routine investigations.

The blood results arrived a few days later. Her Hb was 12.1 g/dL. Her blood group was AB, rhesus negative. The STD screen was negative and she was found to be immune to rubella. Table 8.7 shows the common prenatal tests carried out in pregnancy.

'Triple' or 'Quadruple' screen – combining the maternal serum assays may aid in increasing the sensitivity and specificity of detection for fetal abnormalities. The classic test is the 'Triple screen' for alpha-fetoprotein (MSAFP), β-HCG, and oestriol (uE3). The 'quadruple screen' adds inhibin-A.

What is the basis of these tests? What is the nuchal thickness test?

Trigger box   **Rhesus isoimmunization**

AD transmission.
Maternal anti Rh IgG form due to fetal RBC leakage.
Antibodies cross placenta – fetal haemolysis (erythroblastosis fetalis).
Fetal hypoxia, acidosis, kernicterus, hydrops fetalis.
Second pregnancy (memory cells).
Indirect Coombs' test.
RhoGAM (RhIgG) given for prevention – destroys Rh + cells in mother & prevents sensitization.

Why is folic acid prescribed in pregnancy?
Why is it important to screen for rubella antibodies?
What is the significance of the urine dipstick result?

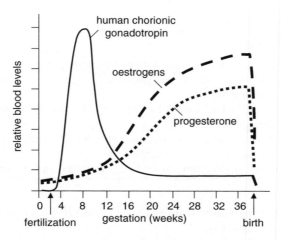

Figure 8.10 Hormonal changes seen during pregnancy. Adapted from Tortora and Grabowski (2003), Principles of Anatomy and Physiology, 10th edition, John Wiley & Sons

The hormonal changes seen during pregnancy are shown in Figure 8.10.

The early peaks in oestrogen and progesterone are produced by the corpus luteum, which is maintained by HCG produced by the chorion. Later, increases in these key hormones are due to production by the placenta. Table 8.8 shows the changes that occur in maternal physiology during pregnancy.

Table 8.8 Maternal physiological changes during pregnancy

Organ/system	Physiological change
Cardiovascular	Increased cardiac output, heart rate and stroke volume. Decreased peripheral resistance.
Cervix	Thick cervical mucus clot expelled at or near labour.
Endocrine	Human placental lactogen, an insulin antagonist, maintains fetal glucose levels. Fetal adrenal glands and placenta produce cortisol. High oestrogen levels increase thyroid-binding globulin.
Gastrointestinal tract	Nausea and vomiting, which is resolved by 14–16 weeks. Increased acid reflux. Constipation.
Haematology	Increased plasma volume and erythrocyte mass. Increased leucocyte count. Increased blood coagulability.
Pulmonary	Increased tidal volume, but decreased total lung capacity, residual volume and expiratory reserve volume.
Renal	Increased glomerular filtration rate. Increased renal plasma flow. Increased aldosterone secretion may cause water retention.
Uterus	Uterus enlarges and palpable per abdomen at around 12 weeks. Displaces the intestines. Irregular Braxton Hicks contractions occur throughout pregnancy.
Vagina	Increased blood flow produces a violet coloration (Chadwick's sign).

Table 8.9 The functions of the placenta

Function	Description
Endocrine	The synthesis and secretion of oestrogens, progesterone, human chorionic gonadotrophin, human placental lactogen, human chorionic thyrotropin and relaxin.
Excretion	Acts as the fetal kidney by disposing of waste metabolites and regulating fluid volume.
Nutrition	Acts as a fetal gut by extracting nutrients from maternal blood and delivering it to the fetus.
Respiration	Acts as the fetal lung by exchanging oxygen and carbon dioxide.

Debbie had further ultrasound scans at 12 weeks' and 20 weeks' gestation. There were no fetal abnormalities detected.

Figure 8.11 shows the development of the placenta.Note the maternal part, the decidua and the fetal part, the chorionic villi. Table 8.9 shows the functions of the placenta.

Trigger box Placental abruption and placenta praevia

Placental abruption
Premature separation of placenta after 24 weeks.
Incidence: 1:100.
Risk factors: Hypertension, trauma, cocaine, previous abruption.
Features: Painful vaginal bleeding; abdominal pain, fetal distress.
Treatment: Expectant management or if serious, delivery.
Complications: Shock; disseminated intravascular coagulation (DIC), fetal hypoxia.

Placenta praevia
Abnormal placental implantation (low lying).
Incidence: 1:200.
Risk factors: Prior Caesarean section, advanced maternal age, prior previa.
Features: Painless bleeding (stops in 2 h), no fetal distress.
Investigations: Transabdominal/transvaginal US.
Treatment: Expectant management, serial US, delivery by Caesarean section.
Complications: Preterm delivery, premature rupture of membranes (PROM).

We can now consider the development of the fetus during gestation. Key developmental aspects involving the systems are covered in the other chapters. For example the development of the nervous system is covered in Chapter 7 and the cardiovascular

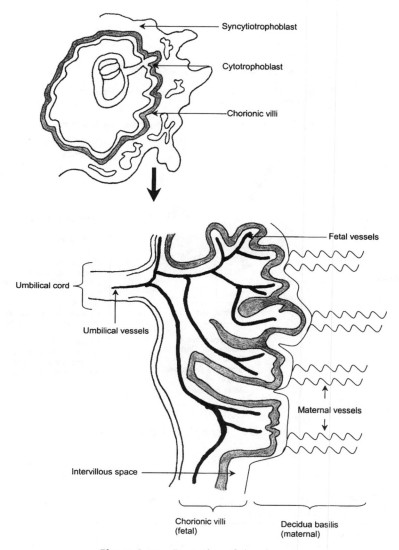

Figure 8.11 Formation of the placenta

system in Chapter 2. Please refer to these chapters for details. Fetal erythropoiesis will be covered in Chapter 9.

Figure 8.12 shows the derivatives of ectoderm, endoderm and mesoderm. Table 8.10 – which you need to complete – shows the important derivatives of the branchial clefts, pouches and arches.

Let us return to Debbie's pregnancy. Her BP during her 32 week visit was 152/92, which concerned the midwife. Her urinalysis showed 1+ proteinuria. She had mild

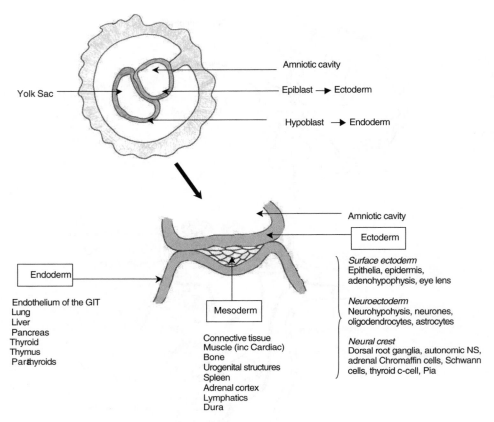

Figure 8.12 Embryological derivatives

Table 8.10 Derivatives of the branchial clefts, pouches and arches complete table. Complete table

Embryological structure	Derivatives
Branchial arch 1	
Branchial arch 2	
Branchial arch 3	
Branchial arch 4	
Branchial arch 6	
Branchial cleft 1	
Branchial clefts 2–4	
Branchial pouch 1	
Branchial pouch 2	
Branchial pouch 3	
Branchial pouch 4	

ankle oedema. She was advised to rest at home and her BP settled to between 138/86 to 146/94. She was seen every week at the antenatal clinic where she had regular CTGs and ultrasound scan every 2 weeks.

 What does CTG mean? What are the different types of deceleration? What is the significance of Debbie's urinalysis and blood biochemistry?

The midwife also visited her weekly at home to check her BP and test her urine. Debbie got very bored at home but she was pleased when Theresa told her every week, 'Your pre-eclampsia is mild and the baby is growing well.'

'I keep my fingers crossed that I'll go into labour before I am induced. Debbie told her. 'I am so scared of the drips and all the messing about in the hospital and I don't want to take any drugs that may harm the baby.'

Trigger box **Pregnancy-induced hypertension**

Aetiology unknown.

Pathology: Vasospasm and endothelial cell damage.

Risk factors: Nulliparity, age <20 or >35, family history, multiple births, renal diseases, chronic hypertension, autoimmunity.

Pre-eclampsia

>20 weeks.

Features: New onset hypertension, proteinuria, oedema, haemolysis, elevated LFT, low platelets (HELLP), oliguria, oligohydramnios, intrauterine growth retardation (IUGR), headache, blurred vision, clonus, hyperreflexia.

Treatment: Bed rest, delivery, hydralazine, labetolol, $MgSO_4$.

Complications: Prematurity, stillbirth, placenta abruptio, DIC, maternal cerebral haemorrhage, aspiration pneumonia, encephalopathy, fetal/maternal death.

Eclampsia

Severe pre-eclampsia + seizures.

Most cases present in the third trimester or within 48 hours following delivery.

Can occur without prior development of pre-eclampsia.

Features: Generalized vasospasm, increased peripheral vascular resistance, haemoconcentration, decreased plasma volume, increased blood viscosity, and coagulopathy. Periportal necrosis, hepatocellular damage, and subcapsular haematoma. Cerebral oedema and haemorrhage, headache, vision problems, seizures.

Treatment: $MgSO_4$, i.v. diazepam, hydralazine/labetalol.

Debbie was also routinely screened for gestational diabetes.

> ## *Trigger box*   **Gestational diabetes**
>
> Around 4% of pregnancies.
> Develops in late pregnancy.
> **Pathology:** Caused by insulin antagonist human placental lactogen (HPL), cortisol.
> **Risk factors:** Age >25, previous macrosomic baby, obesity, family history of DM, stillbirths.
> **Features:** Asymptomatic, polyhydramnios, oedema, large fetus, glycosuria, hyperglycaemia, abnormal OGTT.
> **Treatment:** Diet, exercise, insulin. No oral drugs.
> **Complications:** >50% will develop DM or IGT.
> Hyperglycaemia in first trimester suggests pre-existing DM.

Debbie's concerns...

Debbie had many concerns, and had numerous discussions with the midwife throughout the pregnancy. She was worried about infections that she might contract during pregnancy that might harm the baby. She was also concerned about drugs and other 'poisons' that might harm the baby. She also constantly worried about Down's syndrome. The midwife reassured her and explained that a trisomy was unlikely given her young age. Table 8.11 shows common trisomies.

Table 8.11   Common trisomies

Trisomy 21 (Down's syndrome)
Trisomy 18 (Edward's syndrome)
Trisomy 13 (Patau's syndrome)
Trisomy involving sex chromosomes
XXX (Triple X syndrome)
XXY (Klinefelter's syndrome)
XYY (XYY syndrome)

A trisomy can occur with any chromosome but few babies survive to birth with most trisomies. These trisomies are the most common types that survive without spontaneous abortion.

   Describe the key features of these conditions.

Trigger box   Congenital infections

Toxoplasma
Transplacental transmission.
Also via raw meat, cat faeces.
Features: Hydrocephalus, intracranial calcifications, ring-enhancing lesions on head CT.
Treatment: Pyrimethamine, spiramycin.

Rubella
Transplacental transmission.
Risk very low after 16 weeks.
Screen for rubella immunity. Immunize before pregnancy. Vaccinate at end of pregnancy if titres negative.
Features: Blueberry muffin rash, cataracts, hearing loss, mental retardation, patent ductus.
Treatment: Supportive.

CMV
Most common congenital infection.
Transplacental transmission.
PCR.
Features: Rash, periventricular calcification.
Treatment: Ganciclovir.

Herpes simplex type 2
Intrapartum transmission from active lesion.
Features: multiple, painful vesicles around introitus, dysuria, systemic symptoms CNS, skin, eye mouth infections; neonatal mortality 50%.
PCR, Serology.
Treatment: Aciclovir.

Syphilis
Intrapartum transmission.
Features: Maculopapular skin rash, lymphadenopathy, hepatomegaly, rhinitis, osteitis, sabre shins, sadle nose, Hutchinson's triad.
Dark field microscopy.
Treatment: Benzylpenicillin.
VDRL for screening.

Other infections
HIV, varicella, listeria, malaria, TB, parvovirus.

Table 8.12 shows the key teratogens. Complete the table.

Debbie was also concerned if her baby was growing normally and was relieved when her scan showed normal growth and liquor volume.

Table 8.12   Some teratogens. Complete table

Teratogen	Effects on fetus
Cocaine	Addiction, developmental abnormalities
DES	
13-*cis*-retinoic acid	
ACE I	Renal damage
Iodide	Hypothyroidism/goitre
Warfarin	
Alcohol	IUGR, microcephaly, ASD, maxillary hypoplasia
Folic acid antagonists	
Androgens	
Phenytoin	

Trigger box   Intrauterine growth retardation

Around 5% of all pregnancies.
Fetal weight <10th centile.
Significant discrepancy between fundal height and gestational age.
Types:
Asymmetric (80%): late pregnancy.
Symmetric (20%): early pregnancy.
Causes:
Symmetric: fetal infection, fetal anomalies.
Asymmetric: maternal hypertension, poor nutrition, smoking.
Investigations: Serial US, fetal tests.
Treatment: Steroids, early delivery.

Trigger box   Oligo- and polyhydramnios

Oligohydramnios
Amniotic fluid index <5 (determined by US).
Leads to an increase in perinatal mortality.
Features: Asymptomatic, IUGR, fetal distress.
Causes: Fetal urinary tract anomalies (e.g. renal agenesis, polycystic kidneys), uteroplacental insufficiency, PROM.
Complications: Club foot, pulmonary hypoplasia.
Management: Amnioinfusion.

Polyhydramnios
Amniotic fluid index >20.
Fundal height discrepancy.
Features: Fetal abnormalities.
Causes: DM, multiple gestation, duodenal atresia, tracheo-oesophageal fistula, anencephaly.
Complications: Preterm labour, fetal malpresentation.
Management: NSAIDs (reduces fetal urine output), amnioreduction, steroids.

The birth

The rest of her pregnancy proceeded without major problems. Thankfully, her pre-eclampsia remained mild and she did not have to take medications for her BP. Debbie went into labour one rainy Sunday night. She was in her 37th week of gestation. Max rang the midwife for advice and took her to the delivery suite even before her contractions became regular. The three stages of labour are shown in Table 8.13. Figure 8.13 shows the positive feedback mechanism, which causes uterine contractions. Note the role of oxytocin.

What are the common causes of failure to progress in labour?
Where is oxytocin produced?

Describe the roles of prostaglandin and relaxin in the first stage of labour.

Debbie gave birth to a healthy baby girl by vaginal delivery. Birth weight was only 2.4 kg but she did not have to go to the neonatal unit. Debbie's BP settled to 134/82 soon after delivery but her ankle oedema lasted for another 3 weeks. Table 8.14 shows the key physiological changes that occur in the newborn

The baby's APGAR score at 5 min was 8. What does this mean?

Table 8.13 The three stages of labour

Stage of labour	Event
First stage	(a) latent phase – upto 3–4 cm cervical dilatation.
	(b) active phase– 4–10 cm dilatation (complete).
	Amniotic membranes rupture (naturally or artificially).
	Average duration; nulliparous 8 h; multiparous 4 h.
	Uterine contractions every 2–3 min.
Second stage	Continuing contractions.
	Fetal head descends and completes rotation. Delivery.
Third stage	Delivery of placenta.

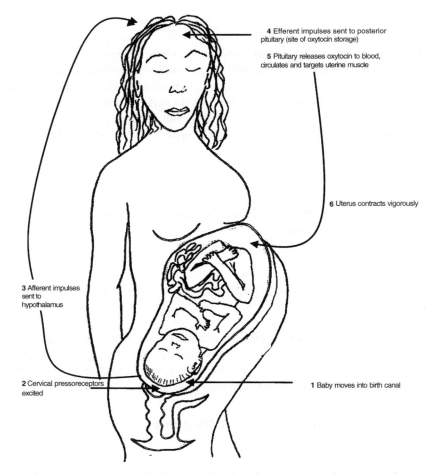

4 Efferent impulses sent to posterior pituitary (site of oxytocin storage)

5 Pituitary releases oxytocin to blood, circulates and targets uterine muscle

6 Uterus contracts vigorously

3 Afferent impulses sent to hypothalamus

2 Cervical pressoreceptors excited

1 Baby moves into birth canal

Figure 8.13   Positive feedback mechanism that causes uterine contractions

Table 8.14   Key physiological changes that occur in the newborn

Change	Description
Cardiovascular	Umbilical arteries and vein constrict. Proximal sections of umbilical arteries form the superior vesical arteries. Pulmonary circulation becomes functional and pulmonary shunts close. The foramen ovale is pushed shut and its edges eventually fuse with the septal wall. Ductus arteriosus constricts.
Respiration	First breath inflates lungs. Alveolar fluid surfactant reduces surface tension.
Nutrition	Reliance on neonatal GI tract to digest colostrum and breast milk. Rapid mobilization of glucose and fatty acids following delivery.
Renal	Development of neonate's kidneys along with increasing glomerular filtration rate. Begin maintenance of acid–base balance.
Thermogenesis	Nonshivering thermogenesis in brown fat to combat hypothermia.

Trigger box   Postpartum infections

1–8% of all deliveries.

Generally polymicrobial. Gram-positive cocci, *Bacteroides*, *Clostridium* spp, *Escherichia coli*.

Risk factors: History of caesarean delivery. Premature rupture of membranes. Frequent cervical examination. Diabetes.

Pathophysiology: Endometritis is the most common source of postpartum infection. In most cases of endometritis, the bacteria responsible for pelvic infections are those that normally reside in the bowel, vagina, perineum, and cervix.

Other sources: Postsurgical wound infections, perineal cellulitis, (*Staphylococcus* or *Streptococcus* spp), mastitis (*Staphylococcus aureus*), retained products of conception, urinary tract infections (UTIs), septic pelvic phlebitis.

Debbie breastfed the baby girl, Susie, fully for 3 months and then only in the evenings and at nights. She had one episode of mastitis, which can occur during breastfeeding.

Trigger box   Mastitis

Cellulitis of periglandular tissue.

Nipple trauma due to breastfeeding, begins 3 weeks postpartum.

Focal tenderness, erythema, purulent discharge.

Staphylococcus aureus (positive milk culture).

Usually unilateral.

Management: Continue breastfeeding, penicillin, erythromycin.

Figure 8.14 shows the reflex mechanism controlling milk production and release. Note the functions of prolactin and oxytocin secreted in response to suckling by the infant.

What are the contents and functions of breast milk?

Which hormones are responsible for breast ductal growth, enlargement of breast alveoli and synthesis of enzymes required for milk production?

Which factor inhibits milk production during the second half of pregnancy?

How does breast-feeding inhibit pregnancy?

Debbie asked Dr Smith when Susie would smile, when she would start crawling and then walking. Dr Smith showed Debbie a chart showing the key developmental milestones. Some of these are shown in Table 8.15.

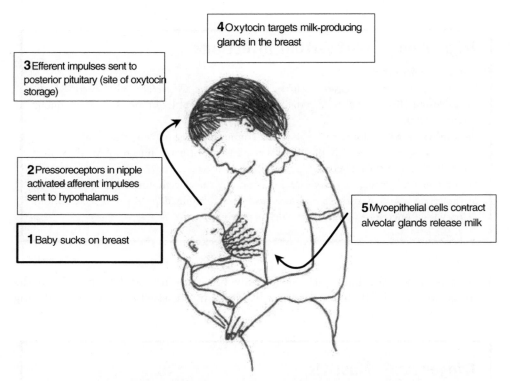

Figure 8.14   Reflex mechanism controlling milk production

Table 8.15   Key development milestones

Age	Abilities
2 months	Social smile, lifts head from prone, parental recognition
6 months	Rolling, sitting, grasping & transferring objects, stranger anxiety
9 months	Crawling, 3 finger pincer, waving, calling to parents
12 months	Walking, 2 finger pincer, imitates
18 months	Use a cup, common words, runs, tower of 3 cubes.
2 years	Jumping, tower of 6 cubes, two-word phrases
3 years	Tricycle, copying circle, 3 word phrases
4 years	Hopping, counting to 10, copying a cross

Mary's changes...

Mary was not at her best. Lately she had begun to suffer from hot flushes, mood swings, was feeling anxious and her mood was low. Her periods had become infrequent in the last one year and eventually stopped six months ago. She also felt vaginal dryness during their now very rare occasions of intercourse. She had an inkling as to the cause of her problems but she went along to see Dr Smith.

Dr Smith checked her age – 52 – and agreed with her diagnosis. 'Yes it looks like you're already in the menopause', he said. He explained that Mary's ovaries had stopped ovulating and were producing less oestrogen as a result. He expected her FSH to be raised but did not feel it necessary to do any blood test to make a working diagnosis. He discussed the management of menopausal symptoms and hormone replacement therapy.

Trigger box **Menopause**

Permanent cessation of menstruation (1 year without for diagnosis).
Ovarian resistance to gonadotrophins.
50–52 years.
Premature (<40) – due to idiopathic ovarian failure.
Risk factors: Smoking.
Findings: Increased FSH, hot flushes, vaginal atrophy, osteoporosis, cardiovascular disease, mood change, dyspareunia, dysuria, decreased breast size.
Treatment: HRT, clonidine, vitamin D, calcium, bisphosphonates, topical oestrogens.

Why is the FSH raised

Describe the advantages and disadvantages of HRT.

Trigger box **Ovarian cancer**

Risk factors: Postmenopausal or prepubescent females, family history of breast/ovarian cancer, nulliparity, delayed childbearing, infertility, late menopause (uninterrupted ovulation).
OCP protective. Why?
Types: Epithelial mainly; germ cell tumours.
Findings: Usually asymptomatic till late – 75% present at stage 3 to 4, abdominal pain, bloating, frequency, vaginal bleeding, weight loss, fatigue, solid fixed pelvic mass, ascites.
Investigations: Pelvic US/CT, CA-125, AFP, LDH, hCG.
Treatment: Surgery (TAH/BSO), chemotherapy, radiotherapy.
Prognosis: 25% 5-year survival.

Trigger box   Breast cancer

Most common cancer in females.

Almost all are adenocarcinomas.

Main histological types

In situ carcinoma (15–30%): Lobular or ductal (80%) carcinoma in situ (e.g. Paget's disease).

Invasive carcinoma (70–85%): No special type (ductal) (80%).

Risk factors: Older age, family history, fibrocystic change with atypia, increased exposure to oestrogen (nulliparity, early menarche, late menopause), *BRCA-1*, *BRCA-2*.

Findings: Hard, irregular painless, fixed lump mainly in upper outer quadrant, nipple discharge, dimpling, ulceration, axilliary adenopathy, metastases in bone, brain, lung, liver. Stage is key prognostic factor.

Positive oestrogen receptor status = good prognosis.

Investigations: Mammography, US, fine needle aspiration (FNA) biopsy, oestrogen/progesterone receptors, Herzneu amplification.

Treatment: Mastectomy, local excision and radiation, axillary node dissection, modified radical mastectomy.

Oestrogen receptor positive – tamoxifen.

Herceptin.

One day several years later Mary presented with vaginal bleeding. Dr Smith referred her to the emergency gynaecology clinic at Hope hospital. He was concerned as post menopausal bleeding is considered to be due to endometrial cancer unless proven otherwise. As it turned out Mary's bleeding was not due to cancer but due to vaginal atrophy.

Trigger box   Endometrial carcinoma

Commonest gynaecological cancer.

Mainly postmenopausal women.

Mainly adenocarcinomas.

Causes/risk factors: Oestrogen: nulliparity, PCOS, late menopause, obesity, tamoxifen.

Findings: Postmenopausal bleeding, premenstral irregularity, intermenstrual heavy bleeding.

Investigations: Ultrasound, hysteroscopy, pipel biopsy.

Treatment: Total abdominal hysterectomy and bilateral salphingo-oophorectomy with or without lymphadenectomy.

Prognosis: 75% 5 year survival.

Combined pill is protective.

9

Genetics, oncology and haematology

Learning strategy

In this chapter we will consider the essential, 'must know' facts and concepts of haematology, oncology and genetics.

A case of colorectal cancer presenting as rectal bleeding will introduce you to the constituents of blood and anaemia. We will discuss haematopoiesis, which would lead to a consideration of leukaemias and lymphomas. A case of thalassaemia will introduce haemoglobin types, heme synthesis and breakdown.

A case of postviral thrombocytopenia will allow discussion of platelet function, clotting and platelet disorders. A haemophilia case will lead on to a discussion of the intrinsic and extrinsic clotting factors and pathways. We will then review the key drugs that target these vital pathways.

We will return to the colorectal cancer scenario to review the key principles of cancer biology and treatment which will allow consideration of DNA structure and function.

This chapter will also provide us with an opportunity to consider the basic principles of inheritance.

Throughout, we will also consider several key relevant conditions and disease states.

Try to answer the questions and try to complete the Learning tasks.

Integrated Medical Sciences by Shantha Perera, Stephen Anderson, Ho Leung and Rousseau Gama
© 2007 John Wiley & Sons, Ltd   ISBN: 978470016589 (HB) 978470016596 (PB)

Albert's bleed...

It is 2004. Things have changed a lot at the bungalow. Albert, now 80, is quite debilitated. His Parkinsonian symptoms are getting worse and he is finding it difficult to cope with his everyday tasks. An outreach care worker had been arranged to help him.

It was the carer who noticed a few spots of blood and mucus on the toilet paper one morning. She took Albert to see Dr Smith along with Mary.

Dr Smith took a history, the questions being mainly directed at the carer and Mary as Albert's speech had deteriorated considerably of late.

Dr Smith ascertained that Albert's appetite had not changed much. A quick weight check confirmed that he had not lost any weight recently. His diet too hadn't changed significantly. His bowel habits however had changed. 'He used to be quite regular' Mary said, 'Just once in the morning, but now he gets constipated then has a run of several a day – he's all over the place'.

Dr Smith examined Albert. He looked a little anaemic but his vital signs were normal. The abdominal examination did not reveal any masses, and there was no tenderness or guarding. Bowel sounds were normal. There were no enlarged nodes and no sign of hepatosplenomegaly.

Rectal examination however revealed a hard mass in the posterior rectal wall and the gloved finger was smeared with blood. Albert was referred to Hope Hospital where a blood test was carried out.

The results are shown in Table 9.1: normal indices are shown within parentheses.

Can you discuss each of these findings?
What are the causes of an increased and decreased MCV?
Why were Albert's serum folate and vitamin B_{12} levels measured?
What is the significance of hypersegmented neutrophils?
What is the ESR? What is its clinical use?

Table 9.1 Albert's results

Haemoglobin	10 g/dL (12–16)
WBC	13.5×10^{-9}/L (4.0–11.0)
Platelets	444×10^{-9}/L (150–450)
Red cell count	2.56×10^{-9}/L (3.00–5.00)
MCV	72.4 fl (80.0–100)
MCHC	288 g/L (320–360)
ESR	79 mm/h (<20)
Vitamin B_{12}	357 pg/mL (187–1059)
Folate	3.5 ng/mL (2.5–11.9)
Iron	5 µmol/L (10–30)
TIBC	90 µmol/L (50–70)
Ferritin	9 ng/mL (15–300)

What is a left shift?
What does a blood film with high levels of reticulocytes signify?

Albert is anaemic and his condition allows us to consider the constituents of blood.

Table 9.2 shows the features and functions of the key blood cell types. Table 9.3 shows the features and significance of several types of abnormal RBC.

Albert's anemia is indicated by a low HCT and Hb relative to the age and gender of the patient. But what kind of anaemia does he suffer from? A scheme of classification of the different types of anaemia is shown in Figure 9.1.

What is the HCT at 2 months of age and in an 18-year-old adult male and female?

Table 9.2 Features and functions of blood cells

Cell type	Main features	Functions
Neutrophil	Lives for 2 days Multilobed nucleus Primary/secondary granules Acute inflammatory cell	Phagocytosis
Eosinophil	Bilobed nucleus MBP, cationic protein, peroxidase	Phagocytosis, antihelminth/protozoa Allergies/parasite infection
Basophil / Mast cell	Granules Mediators (e.g. histamine)	Antiparasitic, allergic reactions
Monocyte	Mononuclear cell In blood for 24 h	APC, phagocytic Precursor of macrophage
Macrophage	Migrates to different tissues	Phagocytic, APC, secretion of cytokines
Lymphocyte	Lifespan long (months/years) Mononuclear cell	Specific immunity (T/B cells) CD4, CD8
Dendritic cell	Found in Mucosa/lymphoid tissue/blood	APC
Natural killer cell (NK)	Large granular lymphocyte	Cytotoxicity, ADCC Tumour surveillance Perforins, granzyme-mediated killing

ADCC, antibody-dependent cell-mediated cytotoxicity; APC, antigen-presenting cell; MBP, major basic protein.

Table 9.3   Abnormal RBC forms. Check these out in a histology text!

Cell type	Disease
Blister cell	G6PD deficiency
Burr cell (echinocyte)	Renal failure, Pyruvate kinase deficiency
Heinz body (this is not a cell type but red cell inclusion body)	G6PD deficiency, thalassaemia, haemolytic anaemias
Helmet cell (schistocyte)	Microangiopathic haemolytic anaemia, artificial heart valves, DIC, post-splenectomy
Spherical cell (spherocyte)	Hereditary spherocytosis, G6PD deficiency, autoimmune haemolytic anaemia
Teardrop cell (dacryocyte)	Myeloid metaplasia, thalassaemia
Target cell (codocyte)	Thalassaemia, haemoglobinopathies, iron deficiency, liver disease, TTP, HUS, post-splenectomy
Mouth cell (stomatocyte)	Hereditary stomatocytosis, liver disease
Spur cell (acanthocyte)	Alcoholic liver disease, post-splenectomy, abetalipoproteinaemia
Oval cell (elliptocyte)	Hereditary elliptocytosis, thalassaemia, iron deficiency
Sickle cell (drepanocyte)	Sickle cell anaemia, haemoglobinopathies

G6PD, glucose-6-phosphate dehydrogenase; TTP, thrombotic thrombocytopenic purpura; HUS, haemolytic–uraemic syndrome.

Albert is suffering from iron-deficiency anaemia.

The iron cycle is shown in Figure 9.2. Iron studies are important in the diagnosis of anaemia. Iron studies in patients with iron deficiency anaemia show a microcytic hypochromic anaemia, with low ferritin (pathognomonic), low iron, increased TIBC and a low percentage iron saturation.

How do these parameters change in anaemia of chronic disease, and thalassaemia?

Other types of anaemia include the megalobastic and haemolytic anaemias.

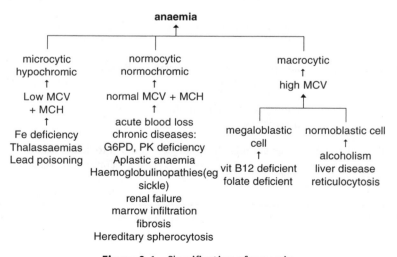

Figure 9.1   Classification of anaemia

Trigger box Iron deficiency anaemia

Most common cause of anaemia.

Causes: Blood loss: menstruation, GI losses, haematuria; dietary deficiency: malabsorption; pancreatic and small bowel disease; increased requirements, e.g. growth, pregnancy.

Clinical findings: Brittle nails and hair, atrophic glossitis, angular dermatitis, koilonychia, pharyngeal webs.

Laboratory findings: Low Hb, low MCV, microcytic, hypochromic RBCs, anisocytosis and poikilocytosis.

Low serum ferritin, low serum iron, high TIBC, low iron saturation.

Treatment: Treat underlying cause

(a)*Oral or parenteral Iron ($FeSO_4$).

(b) Blood transfusion if symptomatic/acute bleed.

*Necessary especially in cases with malabsorption. Oral and parenteral therapy to continue until iron stores replete.

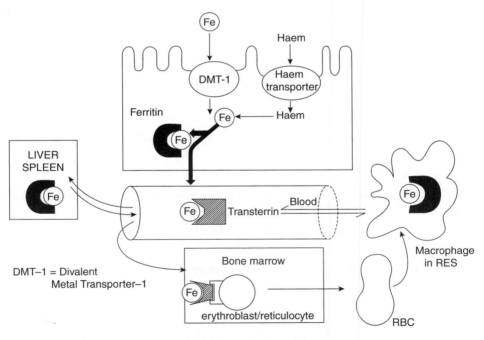

Figure 9.2 The Fe cycle

N.B. DMT-1 transports Fe across apical surface. Haem iron also enters mucosal cell. Fe stoned as mucosal ferritin is lost when cells are shed. Fe is transported bound to transterin. Some Fe stored in liver and spleen bound to ferritin. Macrophages store Fe by breaking down RBCS.

Trigger box Key megaloblastic anaemias

1. *Vitamin B_{12} deficiency.*

Causes: Pernicious anaemia, 'strict' vegans, ileal disease, bacterial blind loop syndrome, drugs (e.g. methotrexate, septrin).

Pernicious anaemia.

A common cause of vitamin B_{12} deficiency.

Failure of intrinsic factor (IF) production.

Elderly, premature greying, blue-eyed women.

Association with thyroid disease and vitiligo (autoimmune disorders).

Features: Glossitis, angular stomatitis, mild jaundice, subacute combined degeneration of cord (weakness, ataxia, visual defects, paraplegia, dementia).

Findings: Increased MCV, hypersegmented neutrophils, low serum B_{12}, low red cell folate, anti parietal cell antibodies, anti IF antibodies.

Increased unconjugated bilirubin.

Investigation: Schilling test.

Treatment: B_{12} injections, Oral B_{12} preparations, which can be used to distinguish between malabsorption and malnutrition by trial therapy.

About a third of B_{12} deficiencies show *no* haematological abnormality. The first presentation could be solely neurological.

2. *Folate deficiency.*

Causes: Poor intake, malabsorption, pregnancy, lactation, prematurity, malignancy, hemolytic anaemia, anti-folate drugs (phenytoin, methotrexate, TMP-SMZ).

Findings: Low red cell folate, increased MCV.

Treatment: Oral folic acid.

In *acute* folate deficiency (following high dose methotrexate), loss can be salvaged by folinic acid rescue or therapy. This is a precursor of folic acid.

Figure 9.3 shows the biochemistry of the megaloblastic anaemias. Note that if there is a deficiency of B_{12}, folate will be 'trapped' in the methyl form. Since folate (FH_4 form) is required for DNA synthesis this key cellular process is inhibited.

What is the most common cause of macrocytosis in the UK?
What is the basis of the Schilling test?

Trigger box Haemolytic anaemias

NB. This trigger box is highly simplified! Try to work out the significance of the trigger words.

Findings: Anaemia, reticulocytosis, unconjugated hyperbilirubinaemia, ↑ LDH.

Intravascular haemolysis: Also methaemalbuminia, haemoglobinuria, haemosiderinuria and reduced haptoglobulin.

Causes:

Inherited

1. *Red cell non-enzymatic syndromes*

Hereditary spherocytosis: AD, common. Ankyrin and spectrin defec[...]
nomegaly, stones, osmotic fragility, splenectomy.

Thalassaemia: see below.

Sickle cell anaemias: see below.

2. *Red cell enzymatic syndromes*

G6PD deficiency: X linked, African, neonatal jaundice, fava beans, quinine, serum enzyme level.

Pyruvate kinase deficiency: Normally young, chronic jaundice from haemolysis. Hepatosplenomegaly.

Acquired

Autoimmune haemolytic anaemia

1. Warm

(Antibody attaches at 37°C).

IgG.

Associated with lymphoma.

Direct Coombs+ve, idiopathic, SLE, methyldopa.

Treatment: High dose prednisolone, splenectomy.

2. Cold

(Antibody attaches <37°C)

IgM.

Direct Coombs +ve, idiopathic, infectious mononucleosis, mycoplasma, viral, lymphomas.

Treat underlying condition.

Paroxysmal nocturnal haemoglobinuria

No GPI anchor; C′ lysis of RBC; progression to myelodysplasia/acute leukaemia; BMT.

Other

Transfusions.

Drugs.

Infection.

March haemoglobulinaemia.

Microangiopathic haemolytic anaemia.

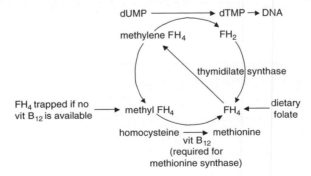

Figure 9.3 Biochemistry of megaloblastic anaemia (FH_4 = folate). Adapted from Howard and Hamilton (1999), Haematology, Churchill Livingstone

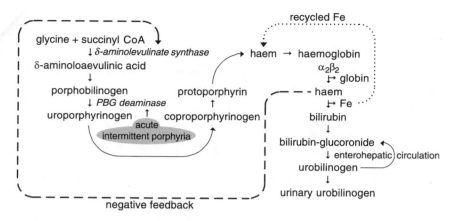

Figure 9.4 Heme metabolism

What is the basis of the direct and indirect Coombs test?

Trigger box Aplastic anaemia

Inherited or acquired (chemotherapeutic agents, chloramphenicol).
Features: Anaemia, infection, bruising, epistaxis, bleeding.
Findings: Pancytopenia low/absent reticulocytes, hypocellular bone marrow.
Investigation: Trephine biopsy.
Treatment: Eliminate cause; transfusions, bone marrow transplant (BMT), antilymphocyte globulin.

Let us now turn to erythrocyte function. Figure 9.4 shows heme formation and breakdown (also explained in Chapter 3). Note the mechanisms leading to acute intermittent porphyria, the most common of the porphyrias.

What is HbF? Compare and contrast its key properties with adult Hb.

Too few RBCs cause anaemia but too many RBCs cause polycythemia.

Trigger box Polycythemia vera

Primary myeloproliferative disease.
Increased RBC production.
Males >60.

Features: Malaise, pruritis, fever, stroke, angina, MI, headache, plethora, large retinal veins, splenomegaly.

Findings: HCT >50%; decreased erythropoietin.

Treatment: Serial phlebotomy, acetylsalicylic acid (ASA), hydroxyurea.

Complications: Increased risk of developing acute myeloid leukaemia (AML), chronic myeloid leukaemia (CML), myelofibrosis.

Secondary polycythemia

Causes: Hypoxia (main), renal tumours, heavy smoking, R–L shunts, altitude, lung disease.

Maria is always tired

On the same day as Albert's appointment Dr Smith had an interesting case. It was a new patient, a 27-year-old Greek woman called Maria. Maria complained of feeling tired all the time. Physical examination did not reveal any abnormalities apart from a palpable spleen. Dr Smith ordered a FBC, and a routine blood chemistry screen.

A week later Maria's results were in. They showed a reduced Hb, a reduced MCV and normal ferritin. All other investigations were normal. Her hypochromic microcytic anaemia, together with her racial background, prompted Dr Smith to order a Hb electrophoresis assay.

 What is the most likely diagnosis?

Figure 9.5 shows interpretation of Hb electrophoretic studies.

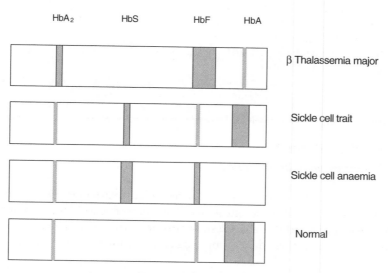

Figure 9.5 Haemoglobin electrophoresis

Maria's Hb electrophoresis revealed a raised HbA2. Maria was suffering from thalassaemia.

Trigger box   **Haemoglobulinopathies**

1. *Sickle cell anaemia*

   AR.
   Blacks > whites.
   Pathology: abnormal HbA β chain, Val substituted for Glu.
   Low O_2/dehydration causes sickling.
   Balanced polymorphism – sickle cell trait.
   Features: Aplastic crises (B19 parvovirus), autosplenectomy, salmonella osteomyelitis, vaso-occlusive crises, infection by encapsulated bacteria.
   HbSC =milder disease.
   Treatment: Hydration, O_2, hydroxyurea, bone marrow transplantation (BMT) (donor type). Blood transfusion. Red cell exchange transfusion.

2. *Thalassaemia*

   (a) Alpha
   Pathology: Underproduction of α chain.
   Asians, blacks > whites.
   Features: HbH, Hb Barts –hydrops fetalis, intrauterine fetal death, chronic haemolytic anaemia, splenomegaly.

   (b) Beta
   Minor – underproduction of β chain – heterozygote.
   Major – Absent β-chain (homozygote).
   Mediterranean, Asian, blacks > whites.
   Features: Increased HbF, bony deformities, hepatosplenomegaly, jaundice, growth retardation.
   Treatment: Blood transfusions (can cause secondary haemochromatosis) along with iron chelation therapy. Bone marrow transplant (donor type).

What is sickle cell crisis?
What is methaemaglobulinaemia?

Let us now consider how blood cells are formed. Figure 9.6 shows the main features of haematopoiesis. Note the pluripotent stem cell that gives rise to all the cells of the blood and the key regulatory factors. Table 9.4 shows the properties of the haematopoietic stem cell. Figure 9.7 shows the sites where embryological and adult haematopoiesis takes place.

  List the current medical uses of haematopoetic stem cells.

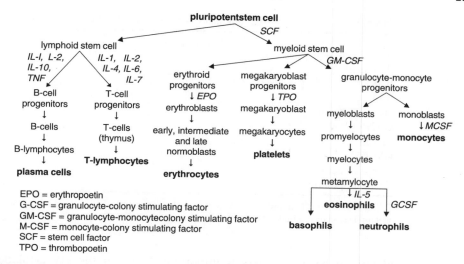

Figure 9.6 Haematopoiesis. Adapted from Kumar and Clark (2006), Clinical Medicine, 5th edition, Saunders

Table 9.4 Features of the haematopoietic stem cell

Undifferentiated
Self renewing
Pluripotent
CD34$^+$
Gives rise to myeloid and lymphocyte pathways

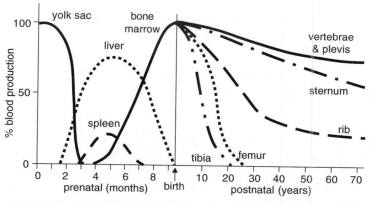

Figure 9.7 Sites of haemopoiesis. Adapted from Howard and Hamilton (1999), Haematology, Churchill Livingstone

Table 9.5   Haematopoiesis: regulatory factors. Complete table

Factor	Function in haematopoiesis
IL-1	
IL-2	
IL-3	
Stem cell factor	
G-CSF	
M-CSF	
GM-CSF	
Erythropoietin	
Thrombopoietin	

IL, interleukin; G-CSF, granulocyte colony-stimulating factor; M-CSF, macrophage colony-stimulating factor.

Precise regulation of haematopoiesis is important. Some of the key cytokines involved in this regulation are shown in Table 9.5. Complete the table.

Which of the above are currently used clinically?
What are the clinical indications of their use?

Regulation of haematopoiesis includes an inbuilt ability to increase the numbers of specific cells when required. For example after a significant haemorrhage or infection, RBC and WBC numbers must be increased. Cytokines are involved in mediating these processes.

Regulation of haematopoiesis also involves programmed cell death, the process of which is termed apoptosis.

What are the microscopic features of apoptosis?

Failure of apoptosis in haematological stem cells and precursor cells can lead to leukaemias and lymphomas.

Trigger box   Leukaemias

1. *Acute lymphoblastic leukaemia* (ALL)
   Malignant cell: e.g. pre B/T lymphoblasts.Subtypes (Ll–L3).
   More in children.
   Features: Marrow infiltration causes anaemia (tiredness, pallor), thrombocytopenia (purpura, petechiae, bleeding) neutropenia (infections with fever), sore throat.
   Lymphatic tissue infiltration: lymphadenopathy and hepatosplenomegaly.
   Other tissue infiltration: bone (limp, bone pain), nervous system, skin.
   Findings: CALLA, TdT, Raised LDH, uric acid.

Treatment: Chemotherapy (good prognosis – 80% cure rate in children). Bone marrow transplant.

2. *Acute myeloid leukaemia* (AML)
   Malignant cell: Myeloblasts: subtypes (M0–M7).
   All ages but less common in childhood.
   Features: Marrow infiltration effects as in ALL.
   Gingival hyperplasia (M5), CNS changes, hepatosplenomegaly, skin rashes.
   Findings: Decreased LAP, Auer rods, myeloperoxidase (MPO).
   Treatment: Chemotherapy, BMT, Retinoic acid (M3) – neutropenic fever, tumour lysis syndrome.

3. *Chronic lymphocytic leukaemia* (CLL)
   Malignant cell: lymphocyte.
   Over 65 years.
   Features: Lymphadenopathy, fatigue, hepatosplenomegaly, warm AHA.
   Findings: Lymphocytosis, smudge cells. CD5 negative. CD19, 20, 22 positive cells.
   Treatment: Supportive treatment, chemotherapy, BMT. Monoclonal antibody (CAMPATH).

4. *Chronic myeloid leukaemia* (CML)
   Malignant cell: myeloid stem cells.
   Features: Asymptomatic, fatigue, fever, splenomegaly, bleeding, blast crisis.
   Findings: Low LAP, Increased vitamin B_{12}.
   Bcr-abl fusion due to ch 9, 22 translocation (T(9; 22))– Philadelphia chromosome
   Treatment: Imatinib (Glivec) >BMT (preferably donor) > interferon >hydroxyurea.
   Poor prognosis: if associated with additional abnormal karyotypes.

Trigger box Lymphoma

Lymphoid tissue neoplasms.

Hodgkin's disease (HD)
Findings: Reed Sternberg cell, single group of nodes, contiguous spread.
Painless lymphadenopathy with/without night sweats, fever, weight loss (B symptoms). 50% associated with Epstein–Barr virus (EBV), hepatosplenomegaly, bimodal distribution.
Most common = nodular sclerosis type.
Treatment: Radiation, chemotherapy (MOPP, ABVD)
BMT. Immunotherapy with CD30 monoclonal antibody and cytotoxic T cells targeting EBV.

Non-Hodgkin's lymphoma (NHL)
Findings: B cells and T cells. Multiple nodes, non-contiguous spread. Painless lympadenopathy, B symptoms, hepatosplenomegaly.

Burkitt's lymphoma
B cells.
T (8; 14) causing c-myc/Ig gene alignment.

Starry sky, EBV, endemic in Africa.

Associated with HIV, immunosuppression.

Age 7–11.

Follicular lymphoma

B cell.

T (14; 18) causing bcl-2/1g gene alignment.

Most common adult lymphoma.

Lymphoblastic lymphoma

T and B cell.

Most common in children; with ALL.

Treatment: Radiation and chemotherapy (R-CHOP). RituxiMab, bone marrow transplant (BMT).

Median survival 3–4 years.

What is the significance of testing LDH, uric acid and leukocyte alkaline phosphatase in the diagnosis of leukaemias?

What is the Philadelphia chromosome?

What are blast cells? Smudge cells? What is a 'blast crisis'?

Little John's scare...

Some years ago there was yet another scare at 10 Sunningdale Avenue. Little John was poorly. The 10-year-old was irritable and was refusing food. He had woken up that morning with a temperature and complained of leg pain and headache. He had also complained that the lights were hurting his eyes. Mary immediately took him to see Dr Smith.

Dr Smith checked his immunizations – Little John was up to date. Dr Smith also asked if he had been in contact with anyone, a child for example who might have had an infection. Mary shook her head; she didn't think so.

Dr Smith began his examination. Little John's temperature was 39.3 °C. His respiratory rate was 32/min. His conjunctivae were inflamed and there was an exudate. His nose was runny. Other than these findings Dr Smith couldn't find anything abnormal. He showed no photophobia and no neck rigidity. 'It's probably a viral infection' Dr Smith said. He advised Mary to give him plenty of fluids and apply tepid sponging for his fever.

Mary returned a couple of days later with Little John. 'He's got a rash' she cried, obviously distressed. 'Oh my God. Is it meningitis? He is complaining of earache and has started coughing'. Dr Smith examined the boy. His temperature was 38.2 °C. He had a rash that was all over his body. 'The rash came on last evening' Mary said. 'It was all

Table 9.6 Little John's results (summarized)

Total WBC	Raised
RBC count	Normal
Hb	Normal
Platelet count	Low
PT	Normal
APTT	Normal

PT, prothrombin time; APTT, activated partial thromboplastin time.

blotchy and started on his face and then spread'. Dr Smith noted a clear chest but red eardrums, inflamed throat and cervical nodes. His eyes and general condition, however, appeared to be better.

Dr Smith reassured Mary. 'Its not meningitis', he said, 'It's a viral infection.'

Mary requested antibiotics. 'Antibiotics will not help.' Dr Smith said. He advised her to keep Little John away from school until he got better. 'I expect him to get better in the next few days. A cold will take a week or so to get better. A proper 'flu will last even longer.'

Mary was back in a week with Little John in tow. She informed Dr Smith that the rash had resolved. His cough and the fever also had gone. But he had developed quite a number of bruises on his legs.

Dr Smith examined Little John. His chest was clear. He noted areas of petechiae on his legs and arms. He phoned the pediatrician on call at Hope Hospital who agreed to see the boy. At the Pediatric Assessment Unit bloods were drawn. The results are indicated in Table 9.6.

The paediatrician diagnosed Little John's condition as postviral thrombocytopenia. He explained that antibodies raised against the viral infection were cross-reacting against his platelets and destroying them. 'It will probably resolve by itself' he explained to Mary. 'But if his platelet count drops below 50, we may have to admit him to hospital for treatment'. 'What kind of treatment? Mary asked. 'Platelet transfusions and steroid treatment, but it is unlikely to happen', the paediatrician said reassuringly.

Little John recovered fully and did not require further hospital treatment.

Trigger box   **Von Willebrand disease (VWD)**

Most common inherited bleeding disorder.

Autosomal dominant.

Pathology: Deficient/defective Von Willebrand factor (VWF), decreased platelet adhesion and factor VIII deficiency.

Features: Bruising, epistaxis, menorrhagia.

Findings: APTT normal or increased.

Treatment: Desmopressin, VWF concentrate, factor VIII concentrate, tranexamic acid.

Trigger box   **Thrombocytopenia**

Platelet count $<150 \times 10^9$/L

Defective production causes

Leukaemia.

Myelofibrosis.

Myelodysplasia.

Aplastic anaemia.

Myeloma.

Megaloblastic anaemia.

Excessive destruction causes

1. *Idiopathic thrombocytopenic purpura (ITP)*
   Autoimmune (antiplatelet autoantibodies)
   Features: Bruising, petechiae, epistaxis, menorrhagia (chronic), afebrile, no splenomegaly.
   Types:
   Acute: In children, post-viral; self limiting.
   Chronic: In adults, idiopathic or with drugs. May be associated with HD and NHL, HIV, CLL, RA, SLE.
   Treatment: Steroids, platelet transfusion, IVIg, splenectomy, immunosuppressives.

2. *Thrombotic thrombocytopenic purpura* (TTP)
   Features: Fever, anaemia, splenomegaly, thrombocytopenia, ARF, seizures.
   Causes: HIV, OCP, pregnancy.
   Treatment: Plasmapheresis, steroids, ASA, splenectomy.

3. *Haemolytic–uraemic syndrome* (HUS)
   Viral infection/gastroenteritis with *E. coli* 0157:H7.
   Features: Anaemia, thrombocytopenia, acute renal failure.
   Treatment: Dialysis.

4. *Disseminated intravascular coagulation* (DIC)
   Pathology: Fibrin deposits in blood vessels due to initiation of coagulation pathway and secondary activation of fibrinolysis.
   Causes: Sepsis, transfusion, trauma, amniotic embolus, neoplasm.
   Features: Epistaxis, hematemesis, hypotension, venepuncture site bleeding. anaemia, thrombocytopenia, increased APTT/PT (consumption of platelets and coagulation factors), D dimers, increased bleeding time, increased fibrin split prods, decreased fibrinogen.
   Treatment: Treat underlying condition, platelet transfusion, cryoprecipitate, FFP.

5. *Others*
   SLE.
   CLL.
   Infection.
   Heparin.
   Drugs.

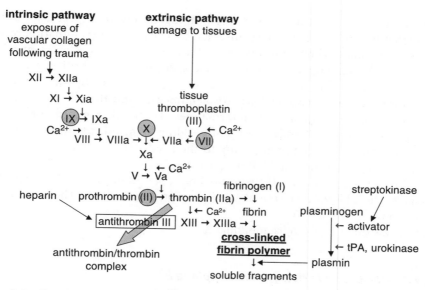

Figure 9.8 Clotting cascade incorporating the sites of action of some anticoagulant and fibrinolytic drugs. Grey circles indicate the clotting factors whose synthesis is affected by warfarin *in vitro*. Adapted from Range, Dale, Ritter and Moore (2003) Pharmacology, 5th edition, Churchill Livingstone

 Find out about. Bernard Soulier disease.

At the Pediatric Assessment Unit Little John's APTT and PT were measured. The APTT and PT measures the factors constituting the intrinsic and extrinsic clotting pathways that are shown in Figure 9.8. Lack of these factors can cause bleeding disorders as seen in the case below. Factors affected by heparin and warfarin are also indicated. The points of action of the thrombolytics are also shown in the figure, which includes the fibrinolytic pathway.

What are the key regulatory proteins acting on the pathway?
What is the function of vitamin K?

Jimmy's big, red, painful knee...

Debbie's friend Sophie called her one afternoon. Sophie was her best friend and lived down the road. She had a 13-month-old baby boy called Jimmy. Jimmy was unwell. He had a developed a swollen and painful knee which had come on suddenly over the past few hours. Sophie mentioned a fall at the nursery earlier that day. She wanted to see Dr Smith and asked Debbie to come along.

Dr Smith took a history. There was nothing untoward expect Sophie mentioning that Jimmy had had some bruises lately. The physical examination revealed a swollen left knee which was tender and warm. The range of movement was restricted. All other joints were normal. He also noted some bruises on Jimmy's legs; they were of different ages. There was no lymphadenopathy. Abdominal examination did not reveal any hepatosplenomegaly and the rest of the systems examination did not reveal any abnormalities. Dr Smith assessed the situation and, especially with the family history of bleeding, concluded that non-accidental injury was unlikely. He referred Jimmy to the paediatrician on call.

At the Paediatric Assessment Unit the doctor ordered some tests. An X- ray revealed no bone injury and showed soft tissue swellings only. Jimmy's blood test results are summarized in Table 9.7a. The raised APTT prompted further tests. The results of these tests are shown in Table 9.7b.

Jimmy was suffering from haemophilia A.

What is the pathophysiology of haemophilia B?
Why was VWF antigen and activity measured?

The paediatrician explained to Sophie that an abnormal factor VIII gene on the X chromosome had led to a decreased production of factor VIII. Because factor VIII was required for clotting, lack of it caused defective clotting and the haemarthroses. This also accounted for the bruising.

Jimmy was given recombinant factor VIII. Later, Southern blot analysis revealed the presence of an intron 22 inversion factor of the factor VIII gene in both Jimmy and Sophie.

Table 9.7 (a) Jimmy's blood results

Total WBC	normal
RBC count	normal
Hb	normal
Platelet count	normal
PT	normal
APTT	raised

Table 9.7 (b) Jimmy's blood results

Factor VIII	low
VWF antigen	normal
VWF activity	normal

Table 9.8 Comparing heparin with warfarin (complete the table)

	Heparin	Warfarin
Mode of administration	Parenteral	
Onset of action		Slow onset
Duration of action	Hours	
MOA	Activates antithrombin III	
Monitoring activity		PT
Overdose treatment	Protamine	

Trigger box **Haemophilia**

X linked recessive.

Pathology: Decreased factor VIII (haemophila A); decreased factor IX (haemophilia B).

Features: Haemarthrosis, intramuscular bleeding, GI bleeding, excessive bleeding from trauma.

Findings: Increased APTT, normal bleeding time.

Investigations: Ristocetin assay.

Treatment: Factor VIII or IX.

How do these lab results differ from those seen in VWD?

? *Patients with protein S deficiency can suffer from DVTs. Can you explain the mechanism?*

Consideration of the intrinsic and extrinsic clotting pathways allow us to study two key drugs that act on these pathways, heparin and warfarin. Table 9.8 shows the main functions of and indications for heparin and warfarin which you need to complete. Table 9.9 shows the laboratory findings in various bleeding disorders.

John's clot busters...

In Chapter 2 we came across John suffering from an acute myocardial infarction. At that time John was treated with thrombolytics, as part of the treatment for his heart attack. John was also prescribed clopidrogel and aspirin. Figure 9.8 shows where in the fibrinolytic pathway these drugs act.

? *Why was John prescribed daily aspirin?*
What is the MOA of clopidrogel?

Table 9.9 Laboratory findings in various bleeding disorders

Increased PT	Increased APTT	Increased Thrombin time	Increased bleeding time	Decreased platelets
Liver disease	Liver disease	Liver disease	Bernard Soulier disease	Thrombocytopenia
Warfarin	VWD	Heparin	Glanzmann's thrombasthenia	DIC
Vitamin K deficiency		DIC	VWD	
DIC	Haemophilia DIC Lupus anticoagulant		Thrombocytopenia DIC	

Construct a table comparing and contrasting arterial and venous thrombosis.

What is Virchow's triad?

Albert has more tests ...

Let us go back to Albert. As we recall Dr Smith referred Albert urgently to Mr Davis, a Colorectal Surgeon at Hope Hospital. Mr Davis carried out an endoscopic colonoscopy and detected an ulcerated tumour 6 cm from the anal verge. The tumour was seen to cover about half of the rectal wall. He also noted three small pedunculated polyps at 30 and 35 cm from the anal verge. There were also several diverticula in the sigmoid colon. He took a biopsy of the tumour for histology and removed the polyps.

What are diverticula? What is the significance of the polyps?

When Albert's pathology report arrived it revealed an infiltrating, well-differentiated adenocarcinoma. He had to have surgery.

What is the significance of the degree of differentiation of the adenocarcinoma?

Mr. Davis ordered more tests prior to surgery. An abdominal and pelvic CT showed no extension of the tumour: the liver, spleen and pancreas looked normal. A transrectal ultrasound examination, however, showed that the tumour had extended beyond the muscle layer. It was within the perirectal fat. Some perirectal lymph nodes also looked infiltrated by the tumour. Surgery and radiotherapy was indicated.

Albert's case allows us to begin our discussion on the biology of cancer. This will require you to initially review Figures 9.9 and 9.10: note the structure of the eukaryotic gene, the processes of transcription and translation. Note how DNA replicates. Complete the table under Figure 9.10.

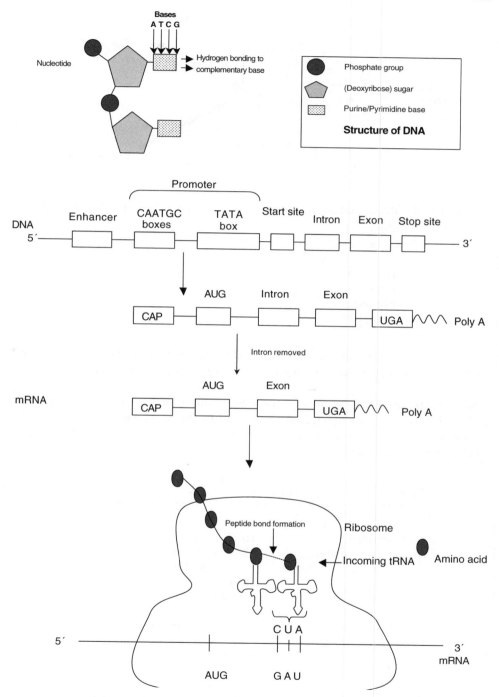

Figure 9.9 Structure and function of DNA: transcription and translation

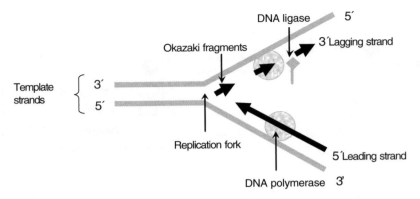

Figure 9.10   DNA replication. Describe the function of the following in DNA replication

Primase
RNA primer
DNA polymerase
Exonuclease
Ligase
Topoisomerase

When reviewing protein synthesis try to figure out the modes of action of key antibiotics that block key stages in prokaryotic protein synthesis.

Colorectal cancer is thought be initiated by a point mutation in the apoptotic gene called APC which causes the mutated cell to escape the normal proliferative controls. Mutations can be chromosomal or single gene. Table 9.10 shows a simple classification of chromosome mutations.

Table 9.10   Chromosomal Mutations

Mutations	Examples
Due to abnormal chromosome numbers	Trisomy 13,18,21 Klinefelter's syndrome Turner's syndrome Mosaicism Polyploidy (e.g.: triploidy, tetraploidy)
Due to abnormal chromosome structures	Deletions: Prader–Willi syndrome, Wilms' tumour, DiGeorge syndrome Duplications: Charcot–Marie–Tooth syndrome Translocations: Down's syndrome

Single gene mutations can result from structural abnormalities (e.g. breakage) in a very small region of the chromosome, or by point mutations within the gene. Point mutations can involve a substitution, deletion or insertion of one base with another. The majority of single gene mutations exhibit mendelian inheritance giving rise to auto-somal dominant, autosomal recessive, X-linked dominant and X-linked recessive patterns of inheritance.

Albert was found to have polyps. In some individuals suffering from an autosomal dominant condition called familial adenomatous polyposis, polyps develop in the colon and rectum and eventually one of these polyps might become cancerous.

In the previous case Maria was suffering from an autosomal recessive condition – thalassaemia – whereas Jimmy's condition – haemophilia- was X-linked recessive. Let us review what we mean by these different patterns of inheritance. Figure 9.11 shows pedigree charts showing inheritance of autosomal dominant, autosomal recessive, X-linked dominant and X-linked recessive traits.

Table 9.11 shows the key AD, AR and X-linked diseases. Find out the lesion and key features of these important diseases.

Mutations could occur spontaneously or be induced by exposure to chemical carcinogens or radiation. DNA damage caused by these agents can be repaired, which must take place before cell division to stop transmission of the mutation to daughter cells. Table 9.12 shows some common carcinogens and the sites of the tumour they induce.

Cells can delay their progression through the cell cycle to allow time for repair. The cell cycle and important control factors are shown in Figure 9.12.

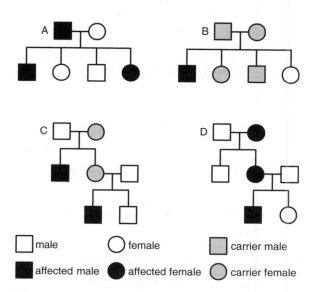

Figure 9.11 Mendelian patterns of inheritance. (A) autosomal dominant inheritance, (B) autosomal recessive inheritance, (C) X-linked recessive inheritance, (D) X-linked dominant inheritance

Table 9.11   Inherited diseases

Autosomal dominant diseases

Achondroplasia	Li Fraumeni syndrome
Alzheimer's disease	Marfan syndrome
Alpha 1 antitrypsin deficiency	Motor neurone disease
Breast carcinoma (familial)	MEN
Congenital spherocytosis	Neurofibromatosis
Dystrophia myotonica	Osteogenesis imperfecta
Ehlers–Danlos syndrome	Polycystic kidney disease
Familial adenomatous polyposis	Retinitis pigmentosa
Familial hypercholesterolaemia	Retinoblastoma
Hirschsprung's disease	Tuberous sclerosis
Huntington's disease	Von Willebrand's disease
Hypertrophic cardiomyopathy	Wilms' tumour

Autosomal recessive diseases

ADA deficiency	Hereditary haemochromatosis
Albinism	Hurler's syndrome
Alkaptonuria	Phenylketonuria
Ataxia telengectasia	Sickle cell anaemia
Cystic fibrosis	Thalassaemia
Dubin Johnson syndrome	Tay Sachs disease
Friedreich's ataxia	Wilson's disease
Galactosaemia	Zellweger's syndrome
Haemolytic–uraemic syndrome	

X-linked recessive diseases

Alport's syndrome	G6PD deficiency
Becker's muscular dystrophy	Hunter's syndrome
Charcot–Marie–Tooth disease	Nephrogenic diabetes insipidus
Duchenne muscular dystrophy	SCID
Fragile X	Turner's syndrome
Haemophilia A and B	

X linked dominant

Rickets (vitamin D resistant)

SCID, severe combined immunodeficiency.

Following cellular damage or DNA damage, cell cycle arrest occurs until the DNA damage can be repaired. However, patients with defects in repair systems cannot do this effectively and thus are more prone to cancer.

 Describe the mechanisms involved in DNA repair.

List the key cancers caused by DNA repair defects.

Colorectal cancer shows multiple genetic changes. Figure 9.13 shows the multistep theory of carcinogenesis as applied to colorectal cancer. Loss of p53 activity results in

Table 9.12 Common carcinogens implicated in cancer development

Carcinogen	Site of tumour
Tobacco smoke	Mouth, pharynx, oesophagus, larynx, lung
UV light	Skin, lip
Radiation	Myeloid leukaemia, skin, thyroid, salivary gland
Alkylating agents	Bladder, bone marrow
Asbestors	Mesothelium in lung
Oestrogens	Breast, endometrium, vagina
Androgens	Prostate
Vinyl chloride (in PVC)	Liver (angiosarcoma)
Polycyclic hydrocarbons	Lung, bladder
Aromatic amines	Bladder
Alfatoxin	Liver
Hepatitis B	Liver
Hepatitis C	Liver
Schistosoma japonicum	Bladder
Human T cell leukaemia virus	Leukaemia
Human papillomavirus	Cervix

cells containing more genetic mutations and chromosomal translocations surviving and being passed on by cell division.

Albert's pathology report revealed an infiltrating, well differentiated adenocarcinoma. Prognosis depends on the histological degree of differentiation of the carcinoma (the grade) and the Duke's stage. Table 9.13 shows what these terms mean.

This brings us to two important types of genes, mutations that could lead to the development of cancer. These are the oncogenes and tumour suppressor genes.

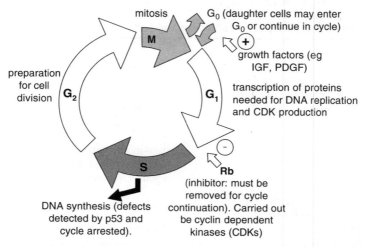

Figure 9.12 The eukaryotic cell cycle. Adapted from Kumar and Clark (2006), Clinical Medicine, 5th edition, Saunders

Table 9.13 Tumour stage and grade

Tumour stage(TNM)		
Example	Ovarian carcinoma	Stage 1 – within ovary only
		Stage 1C – + tumour cells in abdomen
		Stage 2 – within pelvis
		Stage 3 –within abdomen + pelvis
		Stage 4 – Liver & distant sites
Tumour grade	Degree of differentiation	
	Number of mitoses per	
	high power field (HPF)	
	Nuclear pleomorphism	

T, size of tumour; N, nodal involvement; M, metastases.

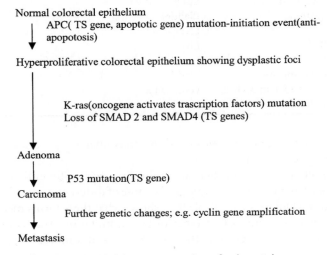

Normal colorectal epithelium
↓ APC(TS gene, apoptotic gene) mutation-initiation event(anti-apopotosis)

Hyperproliferative colorectal epithelium showing dysplastic foci

↓ K-ras(oncogene activates trascription factors) mutation
Loss of SMAD 2 and SMAD4 (TS genes)

Adenoma
↓ P53 mutation(TS gene)
Carcinoma
↓ Further genetic changes; e.g. cyclin gene amplification
Metastasis

Figure 9.13 Multistep progression of colorectal cancer

Table 9.14 Features of oncogenes and tumour suppressor genes

Oncogenes
Mutated pro-oncogenes.
Pro-oncogenes control cell
proliferation and differentiation

Oncogene	**Neoplasm**
bcl-2	Follicular lymphoma
bcr-abl	CML
c-myc	Burkitt's lymphoma
Erb-B2	Gastric, ovarian, breast cancer
Ras	Colon carcinoma

Tumour suppressor genes
Regulate cell proliferation

TS Gene	**Neoplasm**
BRCA 1 & 2	Breast and ovarian cancer
APC	Adenomatosis polyposis coli
RB1	Retinoblastoma, osteosarcoma
P53	50% of cancers

Table 9.15 Paraneoplastic syndromes

Effect	Tumour	Product (if known)
Endocrine syndromes		
Cushing's syndrome	Small cell lung cancer Neuroendocrine tumours	ACTH
Syndrome of inappropriate antidiuretic hormone production (SIADH)	Small cell lung cancer, Intracranial tumours	ADH
Hypercalcaemia	Squamous cancers of lung, breast, kidney and ovary	PTH related peptide
Polycythemia	Renal cell cancer	Erythropoietin
Hypoglycaemia	Sarcoma, hepatoma mesothelioma	Insulin-like growth factor-II (IGF-II)
Thyrotoxicosis (gynaecomastia in men)	Testicular tumours Trophoblastic tumours	β-hCG
Neurological syndromes		
Dementia	Small cell lung cancer	
Peripheral neuropathy	Intrathoracic tumours	
Cerebellar degeneration	Hodgkin's disease Ovarian tumours	
Eaton–Lambert syndrome	Small cell lung cancer	
Dermatological syndromes		
Acanthosis nigricans	Intra-abdominal tumours	
Stiffman syndrome	Thymoma, breast cancer	
Icthycosis	Lymphomas	
Musculoskeletal syndromes		
Finger clubbing	Bronchial carcinoma	
Dermatomyositis	Various	
Haematological syndromes		
Haemolytic anaemia	Non-Hodgkin's lymphoma	

Table 9.16   Key tumour markers

Tumour marker	Tumour
Alpha-fetoprotein (AFP)	Liver, testes
Carcinoembryonic antigen (CEA)	Colon, stomach, breast, lung
Carbohydrate antigen 19-9 (CA 19-9)	Pancreas
Cancer antigen 125 (CA 125)	Ovary
Cancer antigen 15-3 (CA 15-3)	Breast
Calcitonin	Medullary thyroid
Chromogranins	Neuroendocrine
Prostate-specific antigen (PSA)	Prostate
Human chorionic gonadotrophin (β-hCG)	Testes, trophoblastic
S 100	Melanoma,
Neurone specific enolase (NSE)	Neuroendocrine
Paraprotein	Malignant paraproteinaemias (myeloma)
Beta-2 microglobulin (β₂M)	Multiple myeloma and lymphomas

Mutations can appear in oncogenes, genes that normally stimulate cell division or can appear in genes that inhibit cell division, the tumour suppressor genes. Features of oncogenes and tumour suppressor genes are shown in Table 9.14.

Why is the p53 gene called the 'Guardian of the Genome'?

Define the following terms: hyperplasia, hypertrophy, dysplasia, neoplasia.

We can now consider paraneoplastic syndromes. Paraneoplastic syndromes are clinical syndromes that develop in association with neoplasia. These syndromes are not directly caused by the tumour or metastases. Examples of some paraneoplastic syndromes, the tumours, and the products that give rise to the paraneoplastic effects are shown in Table 9.15.

Carcinoembryonic antigen (CEA) can be used to detect recurrences of colorectal cancer after surgery. Table 9.16 shows the key tumour markers used in cancer diagnosis and monitoring.

Albert's main concern is the development of metastatic disease. Metastasis involves the primary tumour breaking through a basement membrane and spreading through the lymphatic and circulatory systems. Metastasis can also occur via the coelomic cavity and the CSF. The most common sites of metastasis are the regional lymph nodes followed by the liver and the lung.

Liver metastases are most commonly derived from colon cancer. Bone metastases are most commonly derived from breast and prostate cancer.

Most common cancers that metastasize are lung and breast cancer.

The most common tumours that metastasize to the brain are lung, breast and skin, kidney and gastrointestinal cancers

Table 9.17 Anti cancer agents

Drug class	Mechanism of action	Example(s)	Cancers treated
Antimetabolites (inhibitors of DNS synthesis)	Folic acid analogue	Methotrexate	Leukaemias, lymphomas
	Pyrimidine analogue	5-fluorouracil	Colon, basal cell
	Purine synthesis blockers	6-mercaptopurine	Leukaemias, lymphomas
DNA damaging	Alkylating agents	Cyclophosphamide Busulfan	NHL, breast, ovary CML
	Non-covalent DNA intercalation	Doxorubicin	HD, breast, ovary, lung
	Cross-links DNA	Cisplatin	Testes, ovary, bladder, lung
	Inhibits topoisomerase II	Etoposide	Lung (SCC), prostate, testes
Antitubulin	Binds tubulin	Taxanes (paclitaxel, docetaxel)	Ovarian, breast
		Vinca alkaloids vincristine, vinblastine	Lymphoma, Wilm's tumor

Albert was treated with radiotherapy and surgery. Some tumours are also treated by chemotherapy. Major anti DNA chemotherapeutic agents and their targets are shown in Table 9.17.

10

Infection and immunity

Learning strategy

In this chapter we will consider the essential 'must know' facts and concepts of immunology and infection.

A case of human immunodeficiency virus (HIV) infection presenting during a pregnancy will introduce you to the immune system. The HIV infection was acquired via the mucosal route and this will lead us to examine some key mechanisms of innate and specific immunity. Viral load testing will introduce the key medically important viruses and antiviral drugs. HIV antibody testing will allow consideration of antibody structure, function and B-cell development.

Several acquired immune deficiency syndrome (AIDS) related infections will allow revision of key pathogens and the principles of systems infection and treatment.

A review of HIV biology and immune responses against the virus will allow us to reflect on the key role of the T helper (Th) cell in mediating immune responses. A discussion of AIDS will lead to a consideration of immunodeficiency. Recalling a transfusion scenario will allow examination of the principles of blood grouping and will lead to the principles of human leukocyte antigen (HLA) typing and mechanisms of transplant rejection.

We will also review the principles of immunization, hypersensitivity and autoimmunity.

Try to answer the questions and try to complete the Learning tasks.

Integrated Medical Sciences by Shantha Perera, Stephen Anderson, Ho Leung and Rousseau Gama
© 2007 John Wiley & Sons, Ltd   ISBN: 978470016589 (HB) 978470016596 (PB)

Debbie goes to the doctors; she is pregnant again!!

Debbie was in the surgery. She was feeling unwell, very tired and low. She was 5 months pregnant with her second child but this tiredness and low mood was new.

Dr Smith took a history, which revealed fever, arthralgia, lethargy, myalgia and a sore throat and headache for the past 2 weeks. He examined her, noting cervical, axillary and inguinal lymphadenopathy. The rest of the physical examination was unremarkable.

Debbie suddenly broke down and began to cry. Max was back on drugs and she was pretty sure that he was seeing someone else. Dr Smith decided to order some blood tests.

What causes lymphadenopathy?

What kind of drugs could Max be using? Table 10.1 shows the features of some common non-prescription drugs.

Debbie's blood results arrived a week later. It showed a lymphopenia with atypical reactive lymphocytes. She also showed a mild thrombocytopenia and her liver enzymes were raised.

What do these results signify?

Table 10.1 Features of commonly used drugs of abuse

Drug group	Examples	Administration	Effects
Group of drugs that reduce pain			
Opioids	Opium	Smoked	Analgesia, anxiety
	Morphine	Sniffed	Contentment
	Heroin	Injected	Higher doses, sedation,
		Swallowed	stupor, and unconsciousness
			Tolerance
			Physical dependence
Group of drugs that alter perceptual function			
Psychedelic drugs	Lysergic acid diethylamide (LSD)	Swallowed	Distortion of perception, feeling of dissociation & 'high', increased appreciation of sensory experiences
Cannabinoids	*Cannabis sativa*	Smoked	Anxiety, panic, talkativeness
		Eaten	Physical dependence less likely
Hallucinogenic mushrooms	*Psilocybe semilanceata*	Swallowed raw, cooked or brewed	Pseudohallucinations (magic mushrooms) Relaxation, drowsiness
Dissociative anaesthetics	Ketamine. Ketalar	Swallowed Snorted Injected	Elation, visual distortion, feeling of floating outside body, nausea, numbness Higher doses like LSD

Table 10.1 (*Continued*)

Drug group	Examples	Admin-istration	Effects
Group of drugs that stimulate the nervous system			
Amphetamines and amphetamine-like drugs	Amphetamines	Sniffed Injected Swallowed Smoked	Increase alertness Diminish fatigue Delay sleep Elevate mood
Tropane alkaloid	Cocaine HCl Cocaine freebase	Sniffed Injected Smoked	Anxiety and nervousness Temporary paranoid psychosis Unpleasant withdrawal symptoms such as fatigue and hunger
Hallucinogenic amphetamines	Methylenedioxy-amphetamine (MDMA)	Swallowed	Effects similar to combining those of amphetamine and LSD
Xanthine alkaloid	Caffeine	Swallowed	Increase alertness
Tobacco	*Nicotiana tabacum, Nicotina rustica, Nicotina persica*	Smoked Sniffed	Diminish fatigue Delay sleep Anxiety and nervousness in high doses
Anabolic steroids	Anabolic steroids (nandrolone, stanozolol, dianabol, durabolin)	Swallowed Injected	Increases aggression and libido Reduce sperm count & quality Non-reversible virilizing effects in women Growth stunting in adolescents
Alkyl nitrites	Amyl nitrite Butyl nitrite Isobutyl nitrite	Vapours inhaled through the mouth	Enhanced sexual pleasure, Rushing sensation, headache, vomiting, dermatitis. Methaemoglobinaemia
Group of drugs that depress the nervous system			
Alcoholic beverages	Ethanol	Swallow	Relieve tension and anxiety, Impair mental and physical function
Minor tranquillizers	Minor tranquillizers (diazepam, chlordiazepoxide, temazepam, nitrazepam etc.)	Swallow	Drowsiness Unconsciousness Decreased self-control Tolerance Strong physical dependence
Solvents and gases	Toluene and acetone (glue) Butane (lighter fuel) Fluorocarbons (aerosols) Trichloroethylene and trichloroethane (cleaning fluid)	Vapours or gases inhaled through mouth or nose	Feeling of dizziness, unreality and euphoria Lowering of inhibition Pseudohallucinations Drowsiness

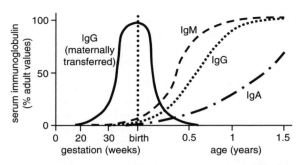

Figure 10.1 Development of immunoglobulin classes. Adapted from Howard and Hamilton (1999), Haematology, Churchill Livingstone.

Dr Smith discussed the results with Debbie. He was concerned about Max's drug habits and gently suggested an HIV test, which she had refused previously. Debbie was shocked. 'Its Max isn't it? She cried. He's been injecting and having sex with all sorts these past 6 months. He's probably given me AIDS hasn't he?'

'Have you had unprotected sex with him since then?' Dr Smith enquired. Debbie nodded.

'What if I have the virus?' Debbie asked. 'Would I have passed it on to my baby?'

Debbie's concerns about AIDS, a disease that, if untreated, systematically destroys the immune system, allows us to consider this very important system. Figure 10.1 shows the development of the antibody response.

 When does the T cell response become fully functional?

Dr Smith noted lymphadenopathy when he examined Debbie. This brings us to lymphoid organs. Table 10.2 shows the primary and secondary lymphoid organs. Primary lymphoid organs are the sites of maturation of B and T lymphocytes where these key cells acquire specific receptors against antigen.

Table 10.2 Primary and secondary lymphoid organs

Primary lymphoid organs	Bone marrow
	Thymus
Secondary lymphoid organs	Lymph nodes
	Spleen
	Mucosal associated lymphoid tissue

Secondary lymphoid organs are the sites where the immune responses against antigen are generated. The spleen deals with blood-borne antigen whereas lymph nodes respond to tissue-borne antigen. Note the important mucosal associated lymphoid tissue.

 Draw longitudinal section drawings of a lymph node and spleen indicating the T- and B-cell regions.

Trigger box **Role of the thymus**

Site of T-cell maturation.

Derived from third branchial pouch.

Rearrangement of T-cell receptor (TCR) genes and expression (RAG1, RAG genes).

Positive selection: Only T cells whose TCR recognizes self major histocompatibility complex (MHC) allowed to survive.

Negative selection: T cells reacting too strongly with self MHC/self peptides destroyed.

Selection takes place in cortico-medullary junction.

Cortex – immature thymocytes.

Medulla – mature thymocytes.

Thymic hypoplasia (Di George syndrome) leads to a T-cell deficiency and hypocalcemia.

What are the other features of DiGeorge syndrome?
Why do lymphocytes circulate?
What are the consequences of a splenectomy?
Where do you find the cisterna chyli? The thoracic duct?

Debbie's results were back. Unfortunately she was HIV positive. The news greatly upset Dr Smith; he had known Debbie since her birth some 25 years ago. Eventually Max too – rather reluctantly – agreed to be tested and was also found to be HIV positive. Stunned by the devastating news Max confessed to Debbie that he had been seeing another woman for the past 9 months, a Zimbabwean hotel worker called Soraya who was seeking asylum in the UK. Worryingly she had had quite a few boyfriends in Zimbabwe. He didn't know her HIV status but they had had unprotected vaginal and anal sex.

It was likely that Max was infected by the HIV virus by heterosexual intercourse. This brings us to consider what happens when the immune system encounters antigen. Initially the innate immune system attempts to clear the virus but if the dose and virulence of the pathogen is high then the specific immune responses are brought into play.

What do we mean by virulence? Table 10.3 shows virulence factors possessed by some key pathogens.

How do these factors enable the pathogen to evade immunity & sometimes cause host damage?

Construct a similar table on viral virulence factors.

Table 10.3   Examples of bacterial virulence factors

Virulence factor	Pathogens
Exotoxin	*Staphylococcus, Clostridium*
Capsule	*Staphylococcus, Streptococcus, Meningococcus*
Protease	*Neisseria, Haemophilus, Streptococcus*
Protein A	*Staphylococcus*
Elastase	*Pseudomonas*
Coagulase	*Staphylococcus*
Endotoxin	*Meningococcus, Salmonella*
Urease	*Helicobacter*
Pili	*Neisseria*

Toxins are important virulence factors: several major infectious diseases such as cholera, tetanus, diphtheria and botulism involve toxins. Table 10.4 shows examples of bacteria that produce toxins and the mechanisms of action of these toxins.

Table 10.4   Bacterial toxins

Bacterium	Toxin	Toxin MOA
Gram +ve exotoxins		
Corynebacterium diphtheriae	Diphtheria toxin	Inactivates EF-2
Clostridium tetani	Tetanospasmin	Blocks glycine
Clostridium botulinum	Botulinum	Blocks Ach release
Clostridium perfringens	Gas gangrene	Phospholipase-disrupts cell membranes
Staphylococcus aureus	(TSST)	Cytokine release
Streptococcus pyogenes	Erythrogenic toxin	Hemolysin
Gram −ve exotoxins		
E. coli	Heat labile toxin	Activates adenylate cyclase; stimulates Cl^- secretion/inhibits Na^+Cl^- absorption
Vibrio cholerae	Cholera toxin	Same as above

The first line of defence encountered by a pathogen is the innate immune system. Table 10.5 shows some innate mechanisms. Try to work out the mechanisms of action of the factors shown in Table 10.5.

Table 10.5 Some examples of innate immune responses

Lysozyme
Complement
Phagocytosis
Cytokines
Acute phase response (e.g. CRP)
NK cells
Anti virals (IFNs α and β)
N.B. IFNs α and β, induced by d/s RNA bind IFN receptor: results in activation of RNA' ase (degrades mRNA) and PKR (inhibits eIF-2)
Binding of IFN-α and -β to NK cells enhances activity
IFNs increase MHC class II activity (how does this help the host?)

NK, natural killer.

What is the acute phase response? What are the key acute phase proteins.

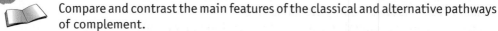

Compare and contrast the main features of the classical and alternative pathways of complement.

Complement is an important innate defence mechanism. Key complement deficiency diseases are indicated in the box.

Trigger box **Complement deficiency diseases**

C1q, C1r, C1s,C4, C2 deficiencies

immune complex disease (systemic lupus erythematosus (SLE), vasculitis, glomerulone-phritis)
recurrent pyogenic infections.

C1 esterase inhibitor deficiency
Hereditary angioedema.

C3 deficiency
severe recurrent pyogenic infections, immune complex disease.

DAF deficiency
paroxysmal nocturnal haemoglobinuria.

Factor D, properdin deficiency
Neisseria infections.

C5b - C9 deficiency
Neisseria infections
SLE.

Table 10.6   Specific immunity. Complete table

Types of response	Mechanism/example
1. *Antibody responses*	
Toxin neutralization	- - - - - - - - - - - -
Complement-mediated lysis	IgM lyses enveloped viruses (classical pathway)
Opsonization	- - - - - - - - - - - -
Generation of inflammatory responses	Activation of complement pathways: C3a, C5a generates inflammatory response
Blockage of attachment	- - - - - - - - - - - -
2. *Cell-mediated responses*	
Tc mediated cytotoxicity	Destroys viral infected cells
Tdth responses	IFN-γ activates infected macrophage

If the innate mechanisms fail to eradicate the pathogen then the specific mechanisms come into play. Table 10.6 shows the components of specific immune response. Note the T- and B-cell responses. Complete Table 10.6.

Figure 10.2 shows antibody functions. Note how binding via FcR enhances phagocytosis (opsonization) and how binding complement can cause lysis of the pathogen cell via the membrane attack complex. Complement activation can also generate C3a and C5a fragments (anaphylatoxins) which, by binding to receptors on mast cells with the subsequent release of mediators (described in Chapter 1) trigger the inflammatory response. Antibodies can also prevent toxin binding and pathogen attachment to epithelia.

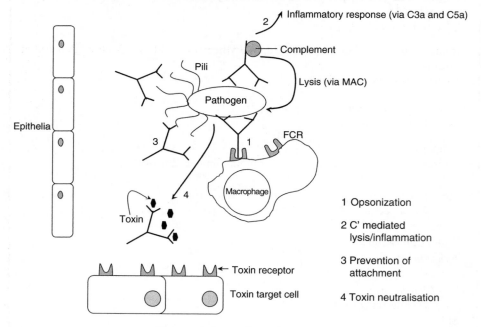

Figure 10.2   Antibody functions

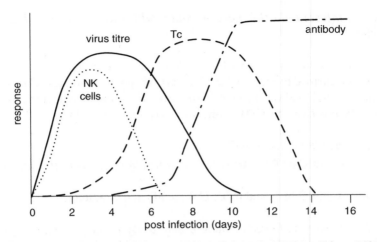

Figure 10.3 Immune response against a typical viral infection. Adapted from Roitt, Brostoff and Male (1996), Immunnology, 4th edition, Mosby

Figure 10.3 shows the immune response against a typical viral infection. Note the initial innate responses (NK cells) and the specific CD8 response that is required to bring down the viral load.

What is the role of antibody in defence against viral infections?
Why is IFN-γ called the specific interferon?

Now let us explore, in more detail, the events leading up to the generation of the specific immune response. Figure 10.4 shows the important process of antigen processing and presentation, which then activate the specific responses. Main antigen-presenting cells include dendritic cells, macrophages and B cells. Note the role of MHC class I and II.

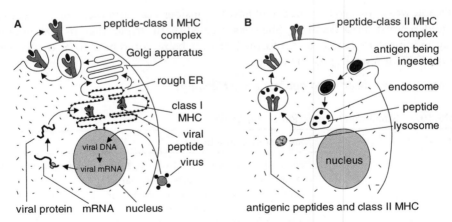

Figure 10.4 Antigen presentation: generation of specific immune responses. 'A' endogenous antigen, 'B' exogenous antigen

If Max was infected via the mucosal route, which APC was most likely to be involved?

Debbie and Max were referred to the HIV clinic at Hope Hospital. Debbie's HIV positivity was confirmed by western blot and particle agglutination tests. Her CD4 count was 870 and her viral load was 1000. All other investigations were normal. Max too was confirmed HIV positive. His CD4 count was 360 and viral load was 12 000.

 How is the viral load measured?
Which cell carries the CD4 marker? What is its significance in HIV infection?

Comment on Debbie's and Max's CD4 counts and viral loads.

 The initial HIV enzyme-linked immunosorbent assay (ELISA) test has high sensitivity and low specificity whereas the western blot shows high specificity. Define the terms sensitivity and specificity, negative and positive predictive value. Is HIV a reportable disease? List the reportable diseases in the UK and USA.

The HIV tests detect anti-HIV antibodies. This allows us to consider the structural features and functions of the main antibody classes shown in Table 10.7 and earlier in Figure 10.2. Figure 10.5 additionally shows how the antibody molecule is generated within the developing B cell. Note the structure of the antibody molecule: the light and heavy chains with the variable and constant regions. Note the structure of the DNA region coding for the kappa light chain containing multiple variable (V), and joining (J) regions. Diversity in the antigen-combining site is in part generated by random combination of a specific V region with a J region in the primary mRNA transcript.

Certain antibodies are important in disease diagnosis. Table 10.8 shows some key diseases diagnosed by antibodies.

Debbie was informed that she might have to consider a caesarian section. She was also advised against breastfeeding. She was treated with triple therapy (zidovudine + lamuvidine + lopinavir) and informed that the baby would have to be treated with zidovudine for 6 weeks postpartum.

Why was Debbie advised against breastfeeding?

Table 10.7 Structure and function of antibodies

Antibody class	Main features/functions
IgM	Pentamer, complement activation, mucosal defense, primary response, first class seen in neonate.
IgG	Complement activation, crosses placenta, secondary response.
IgA	Secretory piece, mucosal defence.
IgE	Mast cell, basophil degranulation.
IgD	Unknown function.

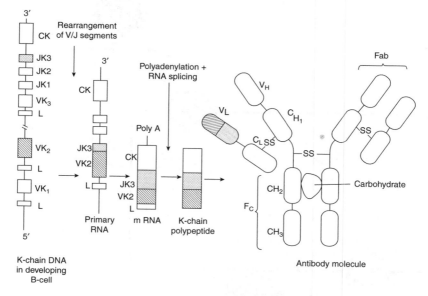

Figure 10.5 Generation of antibody molecule

Let us turn to the virus. Figure 10.6 shows the life cycle of HIV. Note the key molecules, CD4, gp120 and the coreceptor. The coreceptors, CXR and CCR5 are required for entry into the host cell. Note the key viral enzymes reverse transcriptase, integrase and protease; the anti-HIV drug targets.

What are T trophic and M trophic HIV variants?

Figure 10.7 shows the immune and viral parameters in a typical untreated HIV infection. Note the initial viraemia, which is controlled by a strong CD8 response. Note the clinical latency where the viral load is somewhat controlled by a CD4 and CD8 response. Note the slow but steady decline of the CD4 count which eventually leads to a rise of viral load and onset of opportunistic infections and certain

Table 10.8 Some key diseases diagnosed by serology

Rubella
Lyme disease
Leptospirosis
Syphilis
HIV
Gastritis (*H. pylori*)
Hepatitis A, B, C
Pneumonia (*Mycoplasma pneumoniae*)
Chlamydial diseases

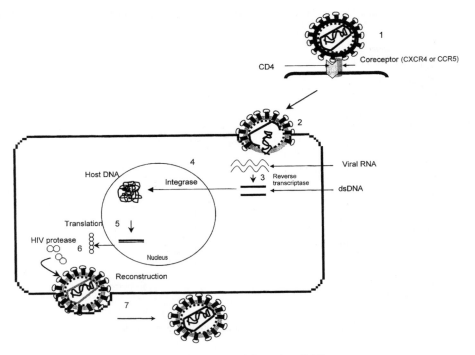

Figure 10.6   The life cycle of HIV

1. HIV GP120 spike binds to CD4 and Coreceptor
2. Fusion with cell membrane, HIV genetic material enters the cell
3. The genetic material of HIV (RNA) is converted to DNA using *reverse transcriptase*
4. The viral DNA integrates into the cellular DNA with the help of *integrase*
5. Viral RNA and proteins are made (*HIV protease*)
6. Viral particles are assembled
7. Virus particles are released from the cell

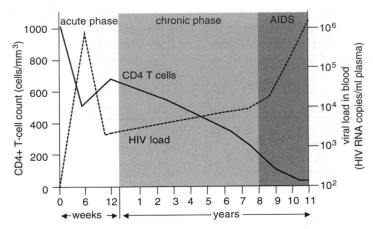

Figure 10.7   Dynamics of CD4$^+$ count and viral load in a typical HIV infection. Adapted from Goldsby, Kindl, Osborne and Kuby (2003), Immunology, 5th edition, Freeman

neoplasms. Note how the parameters change as the patient enters the AIDS phase.

Consideration of HIV leads us to look at the general features of medically important viruses. These are shown in Table 10.9, which you should complete.

What are prions? List the main features of the key prion diseases.

Table 10.10 gives some information about antiviral drugs.

Table 10.9 Medically important viruses. Complete table

Virus	Diseases caused	Key features	Treatment/prevention
1. Key DNA viruses			
Hepatitis B	Hepatitis		IFN α, lamivudine, vaccine
HSV 1 & 2			Aciclovir
VZV	Chickenpox, zoster, shingles		Aciclovir
EBV	Infectious mononucleosis, Burkitt's lymphoma		
CMV			
HHV 6	Roseola		
HHV 8	Kaposi's sarcoma		
2. Key RNA viruses			
Hepatitis A			Vaccine
Hepatitis C			IFN-α, ribavirin
Hepatitis E			
Poliovirus			Vaccine
Rhinovirus	Common cold		
Coxsackievirus			
Rotavirus	Gastroenteritis		
Dengue virus			
Yellow fever virus			Vaccine
Rubella			Vaccine
HIV	AIDS		
Parainfluenza virus			
RSV			
Measles			
Mumps			
Ebola			
Coronavirus			
Influenza			Amantadine, zanamivir, vaccine

Table 10.10   Antiviral drugs

Drugs for herpesvirus infections	Aciclovir, famciclovir, inosine pranobex, valaciclovir
Drugs for cytomegalovirus infection	Cidofovir, ganciclovir, foscarnet sodium, valganciclovir
Drugs for chronic hepatitis B (HBV)	Interferon-α Lamivudine
Drugs for chronic hepatitis C (HCV)	Interferon-α Ribavirin
Drugs for influenza	Amantadine Oseltamivir, zanamivir
Drugs for respiratory syncytial virus (RSV)	Palivizumab Ribavirin

 Describe the MOAs of the drugs mentioned in Table 10.10.

Why is HIV such a difficult virus to eradicate? HIV is able to very effectively evade immune responses by antigenic variation. Table 10.11 shows evasion strategies used by key pathogens. Try to figure out the mechanism involved in each strategy – i.e. how the strategy enables the pathogen to evade immune responses.

HIV infection demonstrates the central role of the CD4 Th cell in mediating immune responses. Have a look at Figure 1.3 in Chapter 1 showing the functions of the Th cell in mediating immune responses. Table 10.12 shows the important properties of the two main Th subsets, Th1 and Th2.

 What is the relevance of a dominant Th1 or Th2 response in leprosy.

Debbie's water works problem . . .

Three weeks later Debbie was back in the surgery. She was now 7 months' pregnant. She complained of dysuria and lower abdominal pain lasting for the past 2 days. Dr Smith examined her. She was apyrexial but her abdomen was a little tender. There was, however, no renal angle tenderness and her uterus was normal size for dates. A dipstick test was positive for leukocyte esterase, nitrite, blood and protein.

 What would renal angle tenderness indicate?
What is the significance of the dipstick test results?

He prescribed amoxicillin and sent off a urine sample for culture. A week later the results returned. Culture revealed $>10^5$ coliforms/mm^3 which indicates infection. Debbie was suffering from a urinary tract infection (UTI).

Table 10.11 Examples of pathogen evasion strategies

1. Viruses

Major structural change in whole molecules of haemagglutinin or neuraminidase of influenza (antigenic shift).

Minor structural change caused by point mutations altering antigenic site on influenza haemagglutinin and neuraminidase (antigenic drift).

Hepatitis C virus blocks action of PKR.

HSV-1 and HSV-2 express ICP47 (expressed shortly after viral replication) which inhibits TAP and blocks antigen delivery to class 1 MHC.

Adenoviruses and cytomegalovirus reduce surface expression of class 1 MHC.

CMV, measles virus and HIV reduce levels of class 11 MHC.

Herpesvirus has glycoprotein that binds C3b.

Direct infection of lymphocytes and macrophages by HIV.

EBV gene homologous to IL-10 (IL-10 suppresses production of IL-2 and IFN-γ).

Low grade infection with persistent shedding, e.g. hepatitis B.

Latency – genome hidden but no expression, e.g. Herpes simplex virus.

2. Bacteria

Proteases secreted by *Neisseria gonorrhoea*, *Haemophilus influenzae* cleaves sIgA at hinge region.

Gene rearrangements of pilin (pili protein) in *N. gonorrhoea* causes evasion of IgA response and increase ability to attach to epithelial cells.

Polysaccharide capsule of *Streptococcus pneumoniae* resists phagocytosis.

Surface M protein of *Streptococcus pyogenes* inhibits phagocytosis.

Coagulase secreted by staphylococci produce a protective fibrin coat.

Long side chains on lipid A of Gram-negative cell walls help resist complement-mediated lysis.

Elastase from pseudomonads inactivates both C3a and C5a anaphylatoxins.

Mycobacteria survive by escaping the phagolysosome.

Table 10.12 Th1 and Th2 subsets and some associated diseases

Cytokine profile	Functions	Diseases
Th1		
IL-2, IL-3, IFN-γ; TNF-β; GM-CSF	Macrophage activation, activation of Tc cells	Tuberculoid leprosy, multiple sclerosis
Th2		
IL-3, IL-4, IL-5, IL-10, IL-13	Antibody production including IgE production, eosinophil maturation, mast cell production	Lepromatous leprosy, atopic diseases

Trigger box   **Urinary tract infection – key facts**

Causes cystitis, pyelonephritis, urosepsis.

Women > men.

Pathogens: *E. coli* (80%), *S. saprophyticus, Enterobacter, Klebsiella, Serratia, Proteus, Pseudomonas.*

Risk factors: Anatomic abnormalities, urinary catheterization, vesicoureteric reflux, benign prostatic hypertrophy (BPH), DM, immunosuppression, pregnancy.

Features: Frequency, dysuria, urgency, fever, back pain, bedwetting.

Urinalysis: Leukocyte esterase, nitrites, including ↑ urine pH, >5 WBC/hpf, >10^5 cfu/mm^3

Treatment: Trimethoprim (avoid in first trimester of pregnancy) nitrofurantoin (avoid in third trimester), amoxicillin, cephalosporins.

Trigger box   **Pyelonephritis**

Infection of kidney.

Same pathogens as in UTI box.

Features: Costovertebral angle tenderness, abdominal tenderness, fever, diarrhoea, dysuria, frequency, urgency.

Urinalysis: WBC casts, leukocytosis.

Investigations: Intravenous urogram (IVU), US in pregnancy.

Treatment: Quinolone, cephalosporins.

Why are women more likely to suffer from UTIs?

Why is *E. coli* ***the most common organism responsible for UTIs?***

We can now consider the main antibiotics used against pathogens. Table 10.13 shows some of the key antibiotics used in clinical practice. Try to find out their mechanisms of action.

Debbie gave birth to baby Zak by caesarian section. Baby Zak was tested for viral DNA by PCR at birth and was found to have HIV. Zak was treated with prophylactic cotrimoxazole for protection against pneumocystis.

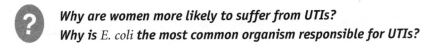

Why wasn't the baby tested for anti-HIV antibodies at birth?

 Describe the principle of the PCR.

Table 10.13 Commonly used antibiotics

Type of infection/ organism	Antibiotic(s) of choice	Alternative antibiotic(s)
Throat infection	None (usually viral)	Phenoxymethyl-penicillin (or erythromycin)
Otitis media	None (usually viral)	Amoxicillin (or erythromycin)
Sinusitis	None (unless severe and >7 days)	Amoxicillin(or erythromycin)
Uncomplicated community-acquired pneumonia	Amoxicillin	Erythromycin
Severe community-acquired pneumonia of unknown aetiology	Cefuroxime + erythromycin ± flucloxacillin	Cefotaxime + erythromycin ± flucloxacillin
Exacerbations of chronic bronchitis	Amoxicillin	Tetracycline (or erythromycin)
Purulent conjunctivitis	Chloramphenicol eye drops	Gentamicin eye drops
Impetigo	Topical fusidic acid	Oral flucloxacillin
Erysipelas	Phenoxymethyl-penicillin	Erythromycin
Cellulitis	Benzylpenicillin + flucloxacillin	Erythromycin
Animal and human bites	Co-amoxiclav	Doxycycline + metronidazole
Septic arthritis	Flucloxacillin + fusidic acid	Clindamycin
Osteomyelitis	Flucloxacillin	Clindamycin
Lower urinary tract infection	Trimethoprim or nitrofurantoin	Amoxicillin or a cephalosporin
Acute pyelonephritis	A cephalosporin	A quinolone
Meningococcal meningitis/ septicaemia	Benzylpenicillin	Cefotaxime
Pelvic inflammatory disease	Ofloxacin + metronidazole	Doxycycline + metronidazole
Uncomplicated genital chlamydial infection or NSU	Doxycycline	Azithromycin
Uncomplicated gonorrhoea	Ciprofloxacin	Ceftriaxone (pharyngeal infection)

Baby Zak gets pneumonia...

At 11 months of age baby Zak began to get sick. He developed severe and persistent diarrhoea. Zak's breathing appeared to be laboured. Debbie also noted white spots in his mouth.

Debbie took him to the clinic where a paediatric HIV specialist examined Zak. His temperature was 38.2 °C and he was tachypnoeic. He also noted crackles in the left lung base. The doctor also noted candida plaques on the inside of the mouth and tongue and around the genitalia. Zak was admitted and bloods were drawn for tests.

His differential blood counts showed a leukocytosis and a reduced CD4 count. His CXR showed left lower lobe consolidation. Zak did not show the expected delayed-type hypersensitivity (DTH) response to intradermal candida antigen or purified protein derivative (PPD). Induced sputum Gram stain and culture revealed *Streptococcus pneumoniae*. Zak was prescribed cefuroxime.

Can you explain Zak's signs and symptoms?
explain the leucocytosis and CD4 lymphopenia?

Baby Zak is also suffering from a *Candida albicans* infection. Key fungal infections are shown in Table 10.14. Complete Table 10.14.

Can you explain the lack of DTH responsiveness to *Candida* and PPD?

The DTH response to candida and PPD is an example of type IV hypersensitivity.

We addressed hypersensitivity in Chapter 1. The pathology of the Type III hypersensitivity reaction is caused by immune complexes. The Trigger box on immune complex disease lists these.

Table 10.14 Fungal infections. Complete table

Fungus	Key features	Diseases caused	Key signs & symptoms	Treatment
Candida albicans	Budding yeast	Thrush, vulvovaginitis, systemic disease, chronic mucocutaneous candidiasis, endocarditis		Nystatin, amphotericin B, clotrimazole cream
Aspergillus fumigatus		Lung aspergilloma, ear infection, invasive disease		
Cryptococcus neoformis		Cryptococcal meningitis, cryptococcosis		
Mucor spp				
Pneumocystis carinii		PCP		

> **Trigger box Key immune complex diseases**
>
> SLE
> Vasculitis.
> Glomerulonephritis.
> RA.
> Serum sickness.
> Cryoglobulinaemia.
> Hepatitis.
> Malaria.
> Trypanosomiasis.

The DTH response can be harmful and is an example of an immune response to infection that can cause host damage. Superantigens, as shown in Figure 10.8 can give rise to an exaggerated DTH response and cause host damage. Staphylococcal toxic shock syndrome toxin is an example of a superantigen.

Other mechanisms of host damage due to immune responses are shown in Table 10.15. Complete Table 10.15.

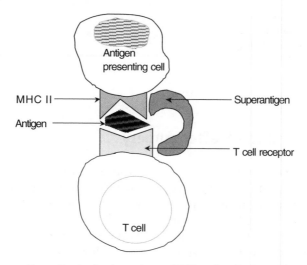

Figure 10.8 Superantigen. Toxic shock syndrome (TSS) toxins (from *Staph. aureus*) may behave as a superantigen i.e. proteins that bind non-specifically to the TCR and MHC II outside of the peptide-binding groove

Table 10.15 Damage to host as a consequence of immune responses (complete the table)

Immune response	Example
1. Production of autoantibodies	
Polyclonal activation	Hepatitis B
Molecular mimicry	- - - - - - -
2. Blocking antibodies	
Antiviral antibody or immune complexes can prevent sensitized T cells from reacting to viral antigens	- - - - - - -
3. Immune complexes	Hepatitis B antigen/Ab complex deposition in arterioles. What causes the pathology?
4. Cell-mediated damage	
Tc cell damage	Rash in measles
5. Inappropriate cytokine release	
	LPS endotoxins from some Gram-negative infections activate macrophages causing secretion of high levels of IL-1, TNF-α leading to septic shock.
	Staphylococcus exotoxin (superantigen) causes similar problems in toxic shock syndrome
	Enterotoxins of *S. aureus* activate T cells causing cytokine release. Responsible for many symptoms of food poisoning – diarrhoea, fever, shock
6. Granuloma formation – tissue necrosis caused by lysosomal enzymes within granulomas	Tuberculosis

Ted gets DIC and ARDS after surgery...

Remember Ted, Irene's brother, who suffers from emphysema? Well he hasn't been doing too well these past few years. His emphysema had steadily got worse. Recently he developed giant bullae in the right upper lobe which occupied nearly a third of the right hemithorax. He was offered a bullectomy.

The operation went well and his immediate postoperative recovery was uneventful. What happened next illustrates another example of how aberrant immune responses can cause serious damage.

Two days later Ted suddenly became confused. The surgeon examining Ted noted pyrexia (38.7 °C), and a thready tachycardia (120/min). Ted's BP was low at 100/72. His WBC count was raised but he was anaemic and thrombocytopenic. He was treated with i.v. colloids, cefuroxime, gentamicin and metronidazole and blood and urine sent for culture.

What could be causing Ted's hypotension and tachycardia?
Why was Ted treated with cefuroxime, gentamicin and metronidazole?

Ted's condition deteriorated over the next day. He drifted into a semiconscious state. His pulse now was 130 and his BP had dropped to 90/45. Arterial blood gases showed a lowered PaO_2 and a raised $PaCO_2$. Ted was admitted to the ICU.

He was suffering from DIC characterized by a coagulopathy, which showed an increased clotting time, thrombocytopenia, and raised D dimers. Classic and alternative complement pathways were also more likely activated.

Why were D dimer levels raised?

Chest auscultation revealed bilateral, widespread crackles. Ted was intubated and intermittent positive pressure ventilation started. Ted was diagnosed as suffering from adult respiratory distress syndrome (ARDS) secondary to sepsis and DIC. Two days later he developed a chest infection and sadly, died.

Trigger box   Sepsis

Septicaemia – systemic inflammatory response to infection.

Gram-positive shock (40%)
Staph./strep.
Exotoxin.
Toxic shock syndrome toxin 1 (TSST 1).

Tampons.

Gram-negative shock (60%)
E. coli, Klebsiella, Proteus, Pseudomonas.
Endotoxin.
Waterhouse–Friedrichson syndrome (meningococci).
Features: Abrupt onset of fever and chills, altered mental status, tachycardia, tachypnoea, hypotension (systolic BP <90).
Starts as warm shock then cold shock (what do these terms mean?).
DIC in 2–3% cases.
Neutropenia, neutrophilia, thrombocytopenia.
Investigations: DIC panel, CXR (may show infiltrates), culture for source.
Treatment: ICU admission, i.v. fluids to maintain BP.

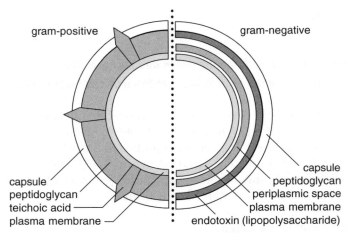

gram-positive   gram-negative

capsule
peptidoglycan
teichoic acid
plasma membrane

capsule
peptidoglycan
periplasmic space
plasma membrane
endotoxin (lipopolysaccharide)

Figure 10.9   The bacterial cell wall

What is the mechanism underlying the pathology of DIC and ARDS?

List the main pathogens causing nosocomial infections

Baby Zak was suffering from pneumonia caused by *Strep. pneumoniae*, an important Gram-positive bacterium whereas Debbie's UTI was caused by *E. coli*, an important Gram-negative pathogen.

Structural differences in the cell walls between Gram-positive and Gram-negative bacteria are shown in Figure 10.9.

Table 10.16 shows some key culture media used to grow bacteria.

Table 10.16 shows the key medically important Gram-positive and Gram-negative pathogens. Complete Table 10.17.

Table 10.16   Culture media

Staphylococcus aureus	Blood agar
Streptococcus pyogenes (group A strep)	Blood agar
H. influenzae	Chocolate with factor V and factor X
N. gonorrhoeae	Chocolate agar
Bordetella pertussis	Bordet–Gengou media
Corynebacterium diphtheriae	Blood Tellurite agar
Mycobacterium tuberculosis	Löwenstein–Jensen agar
Escherichia coli	MacConkey (pink)
Legionella pneumophila	Charcoal yeast extract agar (Fe/Cys)
Fungi	Sabouraud's agar

Table 10.17 Medically important Gram-positive and -negative bacteria. Complete table

Bacterium	Features	Key diseases caused
Gram-positive bacteria		
Staphylococcus aureus	Catalase + coagulase +	
Streptococcus pneumoniae	Catalase −, α-haemolytic	Pneumonia, meningitis, otitis media
Streptococcus pyogenes (gp A)	Catalase −, β-haemolytic	
Clostridium tetani	Anaerobe	
Clostridium botulinum		
Clostridium perfringens		Gas gangrene
Corynebacterium diphtheriae		
Listeria monocytogenes		
Bacillus cereus		
Gram-negative bacteria		
Neisseria meningitidis	Maltose fermenter	
Neisseria gonorrhoeae	Maltose non fermenter	
Haemophilus influenzae		
Brucella abortus		
Bordetella pertussis		
E. coli	Lactose fermenter	
Klebsiella	Lactose fermenter	
Shigella	Lactose non-fermenter, oxidase −	
Salmonella	Lactose non-fermenter, oxidase −	
Pseudomonas	Lactose non-fermenter, oxidase +	

List the main stains used in bacterial identification.

Compare and contrast key clinical features of aerobic and anaerobic pathogens.

Baby Zak was immunized according to the normal schedule. He was, however, given the inactivated Salk vaccine not the live Sabin vaccine. The bacille Calmette–Guérin (BCG) was not given. Zak was additionally given the pneumococcal vaccine at 18 months.

Why wasn't Zak given the Sabin polio vaccine and the BCG?

The current immunization schedule (UK 2006) is shown in Table 10.18. Note the type of vaccine (killed, live, etc.). Vaccines elicit the secondary response via memory cells. Features of primary and secondary responses are shown in Figure 10.10.

What are the advantages and disadvantages of live vaccines?

Table 10.18 UK immunization schedule

Timing	Vaccine(s)	Route	Type
2 months	Polio	i.m.	Inactivated
	Hib type b		Polysaccharide
	Diphtheria		Toxoid
	Tetanus		Toxoid
	Pertussis		Killed
3 months & 4 months	Polio	i.m.	Inactivated
	Hib type b		Polysaccharide
	Diphtheria		Toxoid
	Tetanus		Toxoid
	Pertussis		Killed
	Pneumococcal conjugate vaccine		Polysaccharide
	Meningitis C		Polysaccharide
12 months	Meningitis C	i.m.	Polysaccharide
	Hib type b		Polysaccharide
12–15 months	Measles	i.m.	
	Mumps		Live (a)
	Rubella (MMR)		
3–5 years	MMR	i.m.	Live (a)
	Polio		Inactivated
	Diphtheria		Toxoid
	Tetanus		Toxoid
	Pertussis		Killed
	Pneumococcal conjugate vaccine		Polysaccharide
10–14years*(sometimes after birth)	BCG	i.m.	Live (a)
13–18 years	Diphtheria	i.m.	Toxoid
	Tetanus		Toxoid
	Polio		Inactivated

a, attenuated.

Vaccines should ideally elicit the memory response. What is the basis of this response?

Max is lost to follow up . . .

Shortly after Zak's arrival Max left Debbie and moved in with Soraya. Lost to follow up for 3 years he suddenly turned up at the HIV clinic. He looked rough. He complained of persistent diarrhoea lasting for 3 weeks. His stools were watery and non-bloody. Max also reported some abdominal pain and urgency. He had lost 2 kg since the beginning of his diarrhoea.

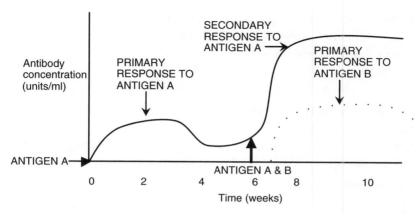

Figure 10.10 Primary and secondary responses to antigen challenge. Adapted from Kuby's Immunology (2000) (WH Freeman and Co)

The consultant began his examination. Max's BP was 116/70, his pulse 92 and regular. He was pyrexial at 37.5 °C. The doctor noted oral candida and palpable nodes in the axilla.

Stool analysis revealed modified acid-fast cysts consistent with cryptosporidia. No acid fast bacilli, amoebae, isospora, microsporidia, or giardia were seen. FBC showed an increased basophil count. Electrolytes revealed low K^+, and Cl^-. The doctor prescribed metronidazole for the cryptosporidium and ketoconazole for the oral candida.

 Can you explain Max's laboratory findings?

Max's cryptosporidium infection allows us to consider some key protozoal infections, which are shown in the summarized trigger box.

Trigger box   **Key protozoal diseases**

NB. You may come across others in different chapters.

Giardia lamblia
Cysts, stool examination.
Foul smelling diarrhoea, bloating.
Metronidazole.

Entamoeba histolytica
Dysentary (bloody diarrhoea).
Liver abscess.
Cysts, stool examination, serology.
Metronidazole.

Cryptosporidium
AIDS, diarrhoea.
Cysts, acid-fast staining.
Metronidazole, Nitazoxanide, Spiramycin

Plasmodia (*P. vivax*, *P. falciparum*, *P. ovale*, *P. malariae*).

Cyclic fever, anemia, splenomegaly, cerebral malaria.

Insect vector: female *Anopheles* mosquito.

Blood smear.

Chloroquine, sulphadoxine, pyrimethamine, quinine, mefloquine.

Trypanosoma (*T. gambiense*, *T. rhodesiense*)

Sleeping sickness, tsetse fly.

Blood smear.

Suramin, melarsoprol.

Trypanosoma cruzi

Chagas' disease.

Reduvid bug.

Blood smear.

Nifurtimox.

Leishmania donovani

Leishmaniasis.

Sandfly.

Amastigotes in macrophages.

Sodium stibogluconate.

Since cryptosporidium is an AIDS-defining illness, poor Max has AIDS. His CD4 count was 180 and his viral load was 225 000. Some key illnesses seen in AIDS patients are shown in Table 10.19.

Table 10.19 Illnesses seen in AIDS patients

Candidiasis
Invasive cervical carcinoma
Cryptococcosis
Cryptosporidiosis
Coccidiomycosis
CMV disease
HIV encephalopathy
Histoplasmosis
Kaposi's sarcoma
Lymphoma
Mycobacterium avium complex
Mycobacterium tuberculosis
Pneumocystis carinii pneumonia (PCP)
Progressive multifocal leukoencephalopathy
Toxoplasmosis
Wasting disease

AIDS is an example of a secondary immunodeficiency disease. Primary immunodeficiency diseases are shown in the triger box below.

Trigger box: Primary immunodeficiency diseases

Complete the table by answering the questions

Disease	Features	Questions
DiGeorge syndrome	T-cell deficiency due to underdevelopment of thymus Tetany, congenital heart defects, recurrent infections	What is the role of the thymus?
Bruton's agammaglobulinaemia	B-cell deficiency, low antibody levels X-linked recessive Defective tyrosine kinase	What are the features?
SCID	B/T-cell deficiency ADA deficiency, MHC 11 failure, IL-2 r defects Recurrent infections	Management?
Wiskott–Aldridge syndrome	B/T deficiency IgM deficiency, increased IgA Pyogenic infections, eczema, thrombocytopenia	Management?
Ataxia–telangiectasia	B/T deficiency IgA deficiency	Clinical features? Treatment?
Selective IgA deficiency	Most common selective immunoglobulin deficiency	Treatment?
CGD	Phagocytic defect – lack of NADPH oxidase Recurrent infections – esp *Staph. aureus*, *Aspergillus*, *E. coli*	Treatment? Function of NADPH oxidase?
Chediak–Higashi disease	AR Microtubular, lysosomal defects of phagocyte Recurrent pyogenic infections	
Job's syndrome	Failure of neutrophil chemotaxis High IgE Cold abscesses by *Staph. aureus*	

CGN, chronic granulomatous disease; SCID, severe combined immunodeficiency.

Table 10.20   AIDS drugs

Type of drug	MOA	Examples
Nucleoside reverse transcriptase (RT) inhibitors	Nucleoside analogues Binds viral DNA inhibiting action of RT. Chain terminators	Abacavir, didanosine, stavudine, zidovudine, lamivudine
Non-nucleoside RT inhibitors	Directly binds and inhibits RT	Efavirenz, nevirapine
Protease inhibitors	Competitive inhibition of HIV protease	Indinavir, nelfinavir, saquinavir

RT, reverse transcriptase.

Max was put on highly active antiretroviral therapy (HAART). Key anti-HIV drugs are shown in Table 10.20.

List the main side effects of these drug classes.

Max gets very sick ...

Two weeks later Max was back at the clinic. He was on HAART but the drugs hadn't had time to start working yet. He had shortness of breath, which had progressively got worse over the past week. He also complained of a dry cough and chest pain and a sore throat with pain on swallowing. He reported losing weight.

Dr Singh, the duty consultant examined Max. He had a temp of 38.2 °C, pulse 103, regular and a respiratory rate of 24/min. His BP was 120/76. He had cervical, axillary and inguinal lymphadenopathy. Pharyngeal examination revealed candida plaques. He had a dry cough and his oxygen saturation dropped to 95 per cent on exertion.

Dr Singh ordered some blood tests. They revealed anaemia, and thrombocytopenia. A chest X-ray revealed bilateral interstitial shadowing. Bronchoscopy with BAL revealed PCP. He was prescribed trimethoprim and sulfamethoxazole (TMP-SMZ).

Can you explain Max's physical findings, blood results and X-ray findings?

Figure 10.11 shows the mechanism of action of TMP-SMZ. Note the synergistic action of these two antibiotics.

Soraya was also sick. She complained of headaches and severe fatigue. In fact she had been feeling unwell for a while now. Max persuaded her to visit the clinic.

Soraya's physical examination showed some focal neurological signs. A lumbar puncture revealed turbidity with a WBC count of 3000/mm³. India ink staining was positive for cryptococcus. She was diagnosed with cryptococccal meningitis, admitted and put on i.v. amphotericin.

Additionally fundoscopy showed signs of CMV retinitis. Soraya was treated with a loading dose of i.v. ganciclovir and oral valganciclovir.

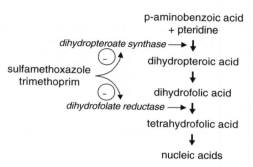

Figure 10.11 Mechanisms of action for sulfamethoxazole and trimethoprim

 Can you describe the main infections of the CNS? Pathogens causing CNS infections and features of the key CNS infections are covered in Chapter 7.

Debbie has a new partner...and a new problem

It was 6 years since Debbie's HIV diagnosis. She had moved on and had a new partner, Mick. She had been fine up until now with her viral loads low and CD4 count high. But today she was at the clinic with a bad case of vaginal discharge.

The consultant examined her. She was afebrile. Her BP was 100/61 her pulse was 90 and regular. There was some axillary and inguinal lymphadenopathy. Debbie's CVS exam was normal. There was also no evidence of hepatosplenomegaly, masses or tenderness. Her neurological exam was also normal. Pelvic examination however revealed a white vaginal discharge but no cervical tenderness. A smear was carried out and the doctor ordered routine blood tests.

Dr Singh noted that Debbie had not attended her yearly smear tests.

One week later Debbie's blood results came back. They revealed anaemia, thrombocytopenia and leukopenia. Her CD4 count was 950 and her viral load was 1100. The cervical smear report came back 3 weeks later. It showed a grade 1 cervical intraepithelial neoplasia (CIN), most likely due to infection with human papillomavirus (HPV).

 HPV infection is an STD. Pathogens causing STDs and features of some key sexually transmitted infections are covered in Chapter 8.

Max's blood transfusion

Remember Max's accident in Chapter 2? At that time he was given a blood transfusion. Let us consider the principles underlying transfusion and transplantation. The main blood groups are shown in Table 10.21. Table 10.22 shows the common complications of blood transfusion. HLA matching in transplantation is shown in Table 10.23. Types of rejection are shown in Table 10.24.

Table 10.21 Main blood groups

Group	Antigen	Antibody in serum	Frequency % (UK)
O(Universal donor)	None	Anti A, Anti B	44
A	A	Anti B	45
B	B	Anti A	8
AB(Universal recipient)	A & B	None	3
Rh +			85

Table 10.22 Complications of transfusion

ABO incompatibility	Clerical error in transfusion is main cause. Immediate reaction. Intravascular haemolysis, rigors, dyspnoea, hypotension. Symptoms 1 week post transfusion – autoimmune haemolysis.
Febrile reaction	Due to antileukocyte antibodies causing pyrogen release. Solution: use leukocyte depleted blood.
Anaphylaxis	Due to anti IgA antibodies in selective IgA deficiency patients. Treatment: i.v. antihistamines.
Infection transmission	Hepatitis B, C, HIV, CMV, EBV, CJD. Test for HbsAg, Hep C antibody, anti-HIV antibody.
Thrombocytopenia	Post transfusion purpura. Develops 1 week post transfusion. Due to antibodies against 1a platelet antigen.

Table 10.23 HLA matching

HLA mismatches	Graft survival after 12 months (approx. %)
None	80
HLA class 1 (1–2 Ags)	75
HLA class 1 (3–4 Ags)	65
HLA class 11 (1–2 Ags)	60
HLA class 11 (1–2 Ags) + HLA class 1 (1–2 Ags)	50
HLA class 11 (1–2 Ags) + HLA class 1 (3–4 Ags)	25

HLA class 11 mismatches have a greater effect on graft survival than HLA class 1 mismatches.
Adapted from T Moen et al. (1980) N Engl J Med 303; 850.

Table 10.24 Transplant rejection mechanisms

Type of rejection	Mechanism
Hyperacute rejection	Antibody mediated (preformed anti-donor Abs) Rejection begins within minutes
Acute rejection	Predominantly cell mediated: (e.g. CD 8^+ activity, vs foreign MHC antigens) Rejection begins weeks after graft Can reverse with ciclosporin
Chronic rejection	Antibody and cell mediated Rejection begins months to years post transplant Fibrinoid necrosis Irreversible

? *How would you manage the situation where there is a reaction due to ABO incompatibility?*

Describe the GVH reaction.

Key immunosuppressants used in medicine are shown in Table 10.25.

? *What are the indications of these drugs? How do they work?*

Table 10.25 Common immunosuppressant drugs

Antiproliferative immunosuppressants
Azathioprine
Mycophenolate mofetil
Corticosteroids(e.g. prednisolone)

Monoclonal antibodies preventing T lymphocyte proliferation
Basiliximab, daclizumab

Calcineurin inhibitors (prevents T-cell activation by new antigen)
Ciclosporin
Tacrolimus

Non-calcineurin inhibiting immunosuppressants
Sirolimus

Monoclonal antibodies causing lysis of B lymphocytes
Rituximab
Alemtuzumab

Epilogue

Dr Smith's last day...

The time had come for Dr Smith to finally hang up his stethoscope and head for his cottage in the country. After almost 40 years of service he was retiring.

He was packing his things in his office. As he glanced around his eyes fell on the card on his bookcase. 'Have a really super retirement' it read. It was from Zoe Sickalott.

Dr Smith sat down and began thinking about the Sickalotts. What a family! What a collection of diseases!

Grandad Albert had finally succumbed to his Parkinsonism, and, not long afterwards Irene too had died of a second stroke. Mary, poor Mary, had never really got over the loss of her parents and John, who had died of a second myocardial infarction at 60. She had been unable to control her drinking and died of liver failure.

Dr Smith shook his head as his thoughts turned to Debbie. Wonder what happened to her, he thought, recalling her HIV status. Apparently she had moved abroad. Then there was Max, with his myriad misadventures, fights, accidents and brush ins with the law. He recalled the phaeochromocytoma, the kidney stone, and finally HIV. He didn't know what happened to Max.

But it was not all doom and gloom. There was one happy ending, one success story: Zoe. In spite of her asthma, and chaotic family circumstances she had somehow managed to get into the local university. After reading law she had secured a good job and was now attached to a top legal firm in the West Country. She had dropped him a line from time to time. Zoe had also taken Little John under her wing, and the lad, from what he had heard, was doing well.

Smiling to himself Dr Smith stood up, picked up his bag and walked out of his office.

Recommended further reading

1. Marks, Marks, Smith (1996). *Basic Medical Biochemistry A clinical Approach* Williams and Wilkins.

2. Sadler (2006). *Langman's Medical Embryology. 10th Ed.* Lippincott Williams & Wilkins.

3. McGeown (1996). *Physiology* (Churchill's *Mastery of Medicine* series). Churchill Livingstone.

4. Kumar & Clark (2002). *Clinical Medicine, 5th Ed.* W.B. Saunders.

5. Kumar, Abbas, Fausto (2004). *Robbins & Cotran Pathologic Basis of Disease, 7th Ed.* Saunders.

6. Tortora and Grabowski (2003). *Principles of Anatomy and Physiology. 10th Ed.* John Wiley and Sons.

7. Rang, Dale, Ritter and Moore (2003). *Pharmacology. 5th Ed.* Churchill Livingstone.

8. Ackland (2006). Ackland's Video/DVD *Atlas of human anatomy, Vols 1–6.* Lippincott Williams & Wilkins.
   (an excellent resource for learning anatomy!)

Integrated Medical Sciences   by Shantha Perera, Stephen Anderson, H Leung and R Gama
© 2007 John Wiley & Sons, Ltd   ISBN: 0-470-01659-6

Index

Integrated Medical Sciences by Shantha Perera, Stephen Anderson, Ho Leung and Rousseau Gama
© 2007 John Wiley & Sons, Ltd   ISBN: 978470016589 (HB) 978470016596 (PB)